PLACING AIDS & HIV IN REMISSION

PLACING AIDS & HIV IN REMISSION

A GUIDE TO AGGRESSIVE MEDICAL THERAPY FOR PEOPLE WITH HIV INFECTION

DAVID SENECHEK, M.D.

Senyczak Publications
SAN FRANCISCO

Cover and illustrations by David Senechek, M.D., Jeanne Koelling

Library of Congress Catalog Card Number: 97-91829

ISBN 0-9657466-0-7
Printed in Korea

For additional copies of this book write to:
Senyczak Publications
P.O. Box 31576
San Francisco, CA 94131-0576
or
www.senechek.com

To the courage and tenacity of people with HIV infection, their partners, and families

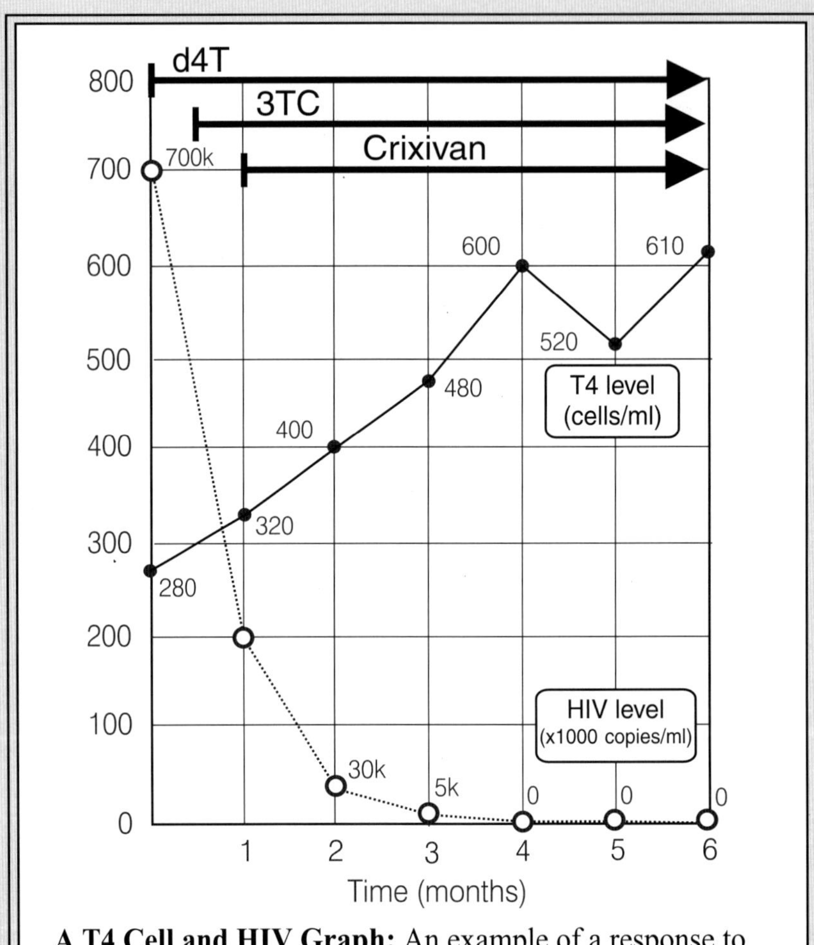

A T4 Cell and HIV Graph: An example of a response to triple therapy. Remission by zero HIV viral level is attained by the rapid addition of d4T + 3TC + Crixivan.

CONTENTS

ABOUT THIS BOOK

Placing AIDS & HIV in Remission is a guide to *understanding* the medical treatment of HIV/AIDS. This book is written to bring simplicity and organization to the broad medical and scientific material in the field of HIV medicine. Much of this material, especially that about viral structure and mutations, is rather complex, but being familiar with this material is crucial to understanding HIV infection and planning rational treatment strategies for this difficult infection.

I've designed the text to cover the history of the epidemic, the structure and life cycle of HIV, and what occurs if one does nothing to stop HIV infection. I've also included a description of the types of medicines available, their positive and negative aspects, and future medicines in various stages of development. The core of the book is about treating HIV with triple and quadruple therapy both for simple and complex cases, with additional chapters on resistance, preventing infections, treating Wasting Syndrome, economics, and the search for a cure.

The book is divided into sections by bold subtitles in each of its 10 chapters with many illustrations to assist the reader to understand or to quickly scan the material for an area of particular interest, if desired.

Finally, this book is not intended to be directive in therapy nor to replace the crucial relationship between doctor and patient. Its purpose is to describe signs and symptoms of HIV/AIDS and provide information to people with HIV, their families and friends, and to medical personnel in the field of HIV therapy. This book is not a substitute for the services of a physician nor is it meant to encourage diagnosis and treatment of HIV disease or its associated medical conditions by the layperson. Proper diagnosis and treatment can only be performed by a qualified physician. No person should initiate therapy or change therapy without the direct, active participation and approval of a physician. It is hoped that this book will help patients and their doctors and medical providers better understand the concepts of HIV therapy so that they can make more accurate and sensible decisions in the treatment of HIV infection.

ACKNOWLEDGMENTS

My thanks for the unwavering support of my business manager and confidante, Carlos Hooks, and my front office manager, Annalisa Delapaz, and for the unlimited support and encouragement of my parents, Robert and Doris Senechek, and my wise friends Mary Rathbun (*Brownie Mary*), Vic and Sissy Riffin, Faye Moore, the Hon. P. A. Bennett, Edwin Hawkins, Sam Sirhed, Pat Brown, and Claudette Amend. My deepest thanks to God for his many blessings, counsel, and teachings.

Special thanks to Dr. Daniel Conlin, Dr. Robert Elsen, Dr. Brian Andrews, Suzanne Wright, Kenneth Coker, Judy and Tia Green, Marcus Wonacott, Andy Pesce, David Lewis, Dr. Jim Const, Ronald Hill, Dr. Rudolf Isch, Tony Siress, Alan Gipson, Dr. Kathleen Kennedy, Irving Gongora, Jeff Morgan, and Elton Bolden, and for the years of support from Martin Delaney, Tom Kelly, and the staff of Project Inform. My appreciation to the staff, associates, and all of my supporters of the Cable Car Committee for honoring me with the Man of the Year Award. My thanks to Judy Ream, Alan Senechek, Jon and Dawn Senechek, Tina Ream, Stacey Ream, Christopher Ream, Brandon King, and the encouragement of Joanne Bender.

It was a pleasure and a great compliment working with Doris Ober who provided the editing to bring this material to a clear and readable format, and with my illustrator and graphics artist, Jeanne Koelling, who translated my drawings into clear design and art form.

I deeply appreciate the support of Harvard University and M.I.T. during my years of study in the Health Sciences and Technology Program at Harvard Medical School. Many doctors and researchers there inspired me to work in the complex field of HIV disease.

Many thanks also to Dr. Kenneth Woeber, Dr. Larry Mintz, and the staff of UCSF/Mt Zion Hospital, Dr. Martin Brotman, Dr. Allan Pont, and the staff of California Pacific Medical Center, and Dr. Stephen Follansbee and the staff of Davies Medical Center. My early research at San Francisco General Hospital could not have been accomplished without the kind support of the staff of Ward 86, Dr. Donald Abrams, and Dr. Paul Volberding.

My deepest inspiration comes from the many people with HIV whom I treat in my clinical practice both in the past and present. Their courage, humor, generosity, faith, and gratitude gives me the strength to seek answers where many times none have previously existed, and the energy to continue pursuing ever improving therapies for my patients.

PLACING AIDS & HIV IN REMISSION

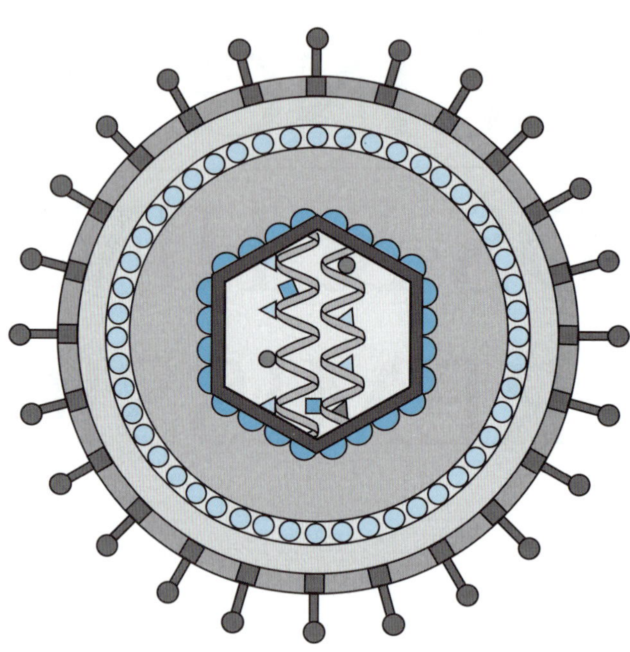

HIV: The Human Immunodeficiency Virus

This unique new life form called a Retrovirus was discovered in 1983 and is the cause of AIDS and HIV disease.

PROLOGUE

In the life of any epidemic, three phases occur:

Phase 1: the discovery of the cause of the epidemic,

Phase 2: the development of effective treatments for the disease,

Phase 3: the cure and the end of the epidemic.

For the AIDS epidemic, Phase 1 was accomplished in 1983 when Dr. Montagnier and his team at the Pasteur Institute in Paris discovered that the Human Immunodeficiency Virus, HIV, was the cause. Although controversy over the mechanism, pathogenesis, and possible co-factors of AIDS raged for more than 10 years, it is now confirmed that HIV is the direct cause of the worldwide HIV/AIDS epidemic.

This epidemic now spans the entire globe, and in the United States it exists in all states and virtually all cities across our land. In the U.S. alone, HIV infects more than one million citizens, has cost the country billions of dollars in resources, and has killed more than 350,000 members of our population. It is now the leading cause of death in U.S. citizens between the ages of 21 and 45.

Treatment for HIV infection has been fraught with failure. National guidelines have instructed physicians to use AZT as single therapy for more than seven years, even though it was widely known that the virus changed or mutated rapidly, and thus bypassed AZT therapy within six months of initiating treatment. These guidelines led to widespread treatment failures, followed by a national hopelessness experienced by both patients and health care providers alike, as hundreds of thousands of people with HIV/AIDS continued to die of the disease.

But a few bold physicians and medical groups within the United States were paying close attention to the basic science data that began emerging in 1990. These data demonstrated the high mutation rate of HIV. By applying lessons learned in the 1950s during the Tuberculosis epidemic (Tuberculosis like HIV mutates rapidly), these physicians moved their patients to aggressive early **combination therapy** with impressive results. As Protease Inhibitors became widely available in 1996, advanced groups moved their patients onto **triple therapy**. The results have been stunning. People on triple therapy typically regain normal health at amazing speeds, while their levels of HIV infection become undetectable, a condition I refer to as **HIV in Remission**. Weight, energy, and daily function return to normal. The medical establishment is watching serious illness disappear among its HIV-infected patients. Hospitalization and death rates are dropping rapidly and show no signs of returning to the numbers seen during the height of the epidemic.

It is clear that we have reached Phase 2 of the HIV epidemic. The year 1996 will go down in history as the year that HIV became a treatable disease. Everyone with HIV/AIDS now has the opportunity to regain normal or near normal health. People who are treated early with aggressive triple therapy by knowledgeable physicians will probably never have to die of AIDS.

So why are so many people in America still suffering and dying of this disease? A look at recent national statistics shows that **only 30% of people with HIV are on any therapy at all.** Of those, most are still on AZT single therapy. It is likely that **less than 5% of people with HIV nationally are on effective triple therapy.**

This book is a guide for both health care providers and people with HIV. Its goal is to translate advanced scientific data on HIV and the disease it causes into an easy to understand, easy to follow system of therapy. With this knowledge, patients and physicians can achieve full HIV Remission in each case. With HIV in Remission, the immune system regains strength, and with simple treatment strategies to prevent infections and reverse Wasting Syndrome, quality of life can return to normal, and the risk of serious illness and death from AIDS can be greatly reduced, even eliminated.

With good information and understanding, people with HIV finally have an excellent chance of living a long life and beating HIV.

1
THE GLOBAL EPIDEMIC EMERGES

1 THE GLOBAL EPIDEMIC EMERGES

And I looked, and behold a pale horse: and the name that sat on him was Death.

--Revelation 6:8

The world was ripe for the development of a new epidemic in the 1970s. By then many in the medical field considered infectious diseases a thing of the past. A treatment and cure had been discovered for tuberculosis, and the polio epidemic had long been eradicated. The U.S. pharmaceutical industry had developed hundreds of antibiotics, and an overwhelming sense of confidence had settled over the land. It was nearly unthinkable that an epidemic could sweep the United States in this era of such advanced science. However, cases of HIV/AIDS had actually begun to occur as early as 1959 in Great Britain and in the 1960s in Central Africa. By the mid 1970s, the disease was spreading rapidly and silently in Africa, Europe, and the metropolitan U.S.

HIV/AIDS IN A BRITISH SAILOR IN 1959

The earliest documented case of HIV/AIDS is that of a 25-year-old British sailor who had traveled to Central Africa in the five years prior to his illness and death. Although he was never married, his lifestyle is unknown. He presented to his doctors in Great Britain early in 1959 with fevers, night sweats, weight loss, and breathlessness. On exam he had large nasal, oral, and anal ulcers. His skin and nails showed signs of fungal infection. On chest x-ray, he had an interstitial pneumonia (a lung infection which diffusely includes all parts of both lungs). Despite treatment for his multiple infections, he died that September. On postmortem PCP (Pneumocystis carinii pneumonia) and CMV (Cytomegalovirus) pneumonia were confirmed. Staph aureus bacteria infection was also found, although the cause of the multiple ulcers eluded the investigators.

This gentleman certainly had an acquired immune deficiency of some type. He had been seriously ill for almost two years. The nasal, oral, and anal ulcers were consistent with chronic Herpes Virus infections, of which in 1959 there was little understanding and no treatment. PCP and CMV pneumonia are two of the most common causes of death in people with HIV/AIDS today, and almost never occur in any other medical illness. The final answer as to whether this British sailor died of HIV/AIDS may never be known, as tissue has not been available for full diagnostic evaluation. But his clinical presentation, type of infections, and travel patterns fit the description of HIV/AIDS and many who have studied this case believe that it is likely the first described case of HIV/AIDS in medical science.

HIV/AIDS IN A ST. LOUIS TEENAGER IN 1968

A second unique case of HIV/AIDS occurred, in retrospect, in a 15-year-old male teenager in 1968 in St. Louis. He presented with brawny penile and scrotal edema (swelling). He was born and had lived all his life in the St. Louis area and was sexually active, although the details of his contacts are unknown. Over the ensuing 15 months, disseminated chlamydia and Kaposi's Sarcoma were found. Pleural effusions (fluid in the lungs) and ascites (abdominal fluid), as well as anasarca (diffuse swelling) of most of his body worsened. On autopsy, his lymph nodes and thymus exhibited profound lymphocyte depletion. Tissue and blood specimens have since confirmed that this young man died of HIV/AIDS. How he contracted HIV is a mystery. Since he had never traveled outside the St. Louis area, it is most likely that a foreign traveler or a U.S. resident who had traveled to Central Africa and became infected with HIV/AIDS passed the infection to the St. Louis teenager through sexual contact.

AN EPIDEMIC IS LIKE A FOREST FIRE

It starts with a few sparks, many of which burn out without notice. HIV/AIDS may have been occurring in Central Africa for many decades in sporadic small outbreaks. The British sailor and the St. Louis teenager may have represented "sparks" of HIV/AIDS that were not strong enough to become the epidemic we are currently fighting. Only when the environment is just right in many aspects does a spark cause a small conflagration which can become a raging forest fire. Epidemics are frequently preceded by individual cases that "burn out," as these two cases did.

Socially, it was not until the urbanization and destruction of the tropical forests in Central Africa that we began to see new infections emerge from this area. As forests were torn down, animals had to find new situations for food and survival. Green monkeys and other animals began living within the fractured tribal groups of the area. It is likely that through some social interaction, the green monkey, which carries a similar virus to HIV called SIV (Simian Immunodeficiency Virus), passed SIV to humans. Over time, SIV mutated to a more lethal form which we call HIV.

As tribal groups broke apart in Central Africa, men began traveling to the cities to find work. Some women in need of money and food began working as prostitutes for the displaced men. With HIV present in sporadic cases, and its main transmission being sexual intercourse, the epidemic began to spread through the urban areas of Central Africa in the late 1960s and early and mid 1970s.

It is clear now that the current HIV epidemic began in Central Africa. Then approximately five years after HIV was entrenched there, it began traveling to other parts of the world. During this same period, the newly liberated gay or homosexual communities in the U.S. and Europe began traveling too. HIV's transmission to the West centered clearly in and around cities with a well traveled population and where the gay movement was most established, New York, Newark, Miami, Houston, Los Angeles, and San Francisco. One gay Canadian airline steward is believed to have contributed mightily to advancing the disease in those American cities. He was dubbed "Patient Zero," for being the sexual common denominator among at least 100 of the first identified HIV/AIDS cases in the United States epidemic. He died of HIV/AIDS in the early 1980s.

THE CHRONOLOGY OF THE HIV/AIDS EPIDEMIC

Historical data is limited, but the epidemic appears to have progressed somewhat according to the following chronology:

1959 - stored blood from Zaire shows evidence of infection by HIV. A possible case of AIDS occurs in Great Britain.

1968 - increasing rates of infection in Central Africa. A case of HIV/AIDS occurs in St. Louis, Missouri.

1976 - a number of European health care workers who had worked in Zaire and other Central African countries die of PCP and AIDS.

1978 - Five AIDS cases occur in France and three in the U.S. with links to Central Africa and Haiti.

1981 - AIDS is recognized as a new disease. The AIDS epidemic begins.

1983 - The Human Immunodeficiency Virus (HIV) is discovered as the cause of AIDS.

1986 - AZT (Retrovir) is approved as the first medication to treat people with AIDS on a limited basis.

1988 - The number of deaths due to HIV/AIDS exceeds 50,000, surpassing the number of deaths of U.S. personnel in the Vietnam conflict. Governmental and public support is almost nonexistent.

1990 - Data on the mutagenicity of HIV becomes available. National policy continues to recommend no treatment for most with HIV, and limited AZT single therapy for those with Advanced HIV or AIDS only. A small number of physicians advance their patients to combination therapy despite conservative national guidelines.

1996 - Protease Inhibitors become widely available. The International AIDS Conference endorses aggressive, early combination therapy, and recommends against use of AZT as single therapy.

THE FIRST OFFICIAL REPORT OF AIDS

Dr. Michael Gottlieb was the first doctor to recognize and report that a new disease was occurring in the patients he was caring for in 1980. During a time when the Gay Liberation Movement was in full swing, Dr. Gottlieb began noticing a pattern of unusual illness in young gay men seeking his care in Los Angeles, California. As the numbers of people with this mysterious illness mounted, he wrote the first description of HIV/AIDS in the Morbidity and Mortality World Report in June 1981 [*see Figure 1*].

Little did Dr. Gottlieb realize at the time that he was documenting the first recognized cases of a viral epidemic that would span the globe in less than 10 years, kill millions of people, and devastate the economies of many developing nations.

THE NEW DISEASE IS NAMED GRID

For lack of another more scientific term, the new disease syndrome was initially named GRID for Gay Related Immune Disorder. Theories were rampant as to the cause of this illness. Life style, drug use, Cytomegalovirus, and the wrath of God were ideas that were hotly debated. But none of these explained the new cases being reported every month in babies, hemophiliacs, people receiving blood transfusions, and heterosexual men and women. It soon became apparent that this new epidemic was spread by sexual relations, and blood contamination.

Figure 1 The First Reported Cases of HIV/AIDS in the U.S.

Pneumocystis Pneumonia - Los Angeles

In the period October 1980-1981, 5 young men, all active homosexuals, were treated for biopsy-confirmed Pneumocystis carinii pneumonia at 3 different hospitals in Los Angeles, California. Two of the patients died. All 5 patients had laboratory-confirmed previous or current cytomegalovirus (CMV) infection and candidal mucosal infection. Cases of these patients follow.

Patient 1: A previously healthy 33-year-old man developed P. carinii pneumonia and oral mucosal candidiasis in March 1981 after a 2-month history of fever associated with elevated liver enzymes, leukopenia, and CMV viruria. The serum complement-fixation CMV titer [level] in October 1980 was 256, in May 1981 it was 32. The patient's condition deteriorated despite courses of treatment with trimethoprim-sulfamethoxazole (TMP/SMX), pentamidine, and acyclovir. He died May 3, and postmortem examination showed residual P. carinii and CMV pneumonia, but no evidence of neoplasia.

Patient 2: A previously healthy 30-year-old man developed P. carinii pneumonia in April 1981 after a 5-month history of fever each day and of elevated liver-function tests. CMV viruria, and documented seroconversion to CMV, i.e., an acute-phase titer of 16 and features of his illness included leukopenia and mucosal candidiasis. His pneumonia responded to a course of intravenous TMP/SMX, but, as of the latest reports, he continues to have a fever each day.

Patient 3: A 30-year-old man was well until January 1981 when he developed esophageal and oral candidiasis that responded to Amphotericin B treatment. He was hospitalized in February 1981 for P. carinii pneumonia that responded to oral TMP/SMX. His esophageal candidiasis recurred after the pneumonia was diagnosed, and he was again given Amphotericin B. The CMV complement-fixation titer in March 1981 was 8. Material from an esophageal biopsy was positive for CMV.

Patient 4: A 29-year-old man developed P. carinii pneumonia in February 1981. He had Hodgkin's disease 3 years earlier, but had been successfully treated with radiation therapy alone. He did not improve after being given intravenous TMP/SMX and corticosteriods and died in March. Postmortem examination showed no evidence of Hodgkin's disease, but P. carinii and CMV were found in lung tissue.

Patient 5: A previously healthy 36-year-old man with clinically diagnosed CMV infection in September 1980 was seen in April 1981 because of a 4-month history of fever, dyspnea, and cough. On admission he was found to have P. carinii pneumonia, oral candidiasis, and CMV retinitis. A complement-fixation CMV titer in April 1981 was 128. The patient has been treated with 2 short courses of TMP/SMX that have been limited because of sulfa-induced neutropenia. He is being treated for candidiasis with topical nystatin.

The diagnosis of Pneumocystis pneumonia was confirmed for all 5 patients antemortem by closed or open lung biopsy. The patients did not know each other and had no known common contacts or knowledge of sexual partners who had similar illnesses. The 5 did not have comparable histories of sexually transmitted disease. Four had serologic evidence of past hepatitis B infection but had no evidence of current hepatitis B surface antigen. Two of the 5 reported having frequent homosexual contacts with various partners. All 5 reported using inhalant drugs, and 1 reported parenteral [intravenous] drug abuse. Three patients had profoundly depressed numbers of thymus-dependent lymphocyte cells and profoundly depressed in vitro proliferative responses to mitogens and antigens. Lymphocyte studies were not performed on the other 2 patients.

More than 80% of the cases worldwide were heterosexual with an equal distribution in both men and women. Only in Europe and the United States were the statistics weighted toward homosexual lifestyle.

REPORTS MOUNT

As the number of cases and the death toll quickly mounted, the Centers of Disease Control alerted physicians and health care workers across the U.S. of a probable mounting epidemic. Three previously unreported AIDS cases had occurred in the U.S. in 1978 and 19 cases were reported in 1979. By the end of 1981, 394 total AIDS cases had been reported. Although small in number, the trend was that of an early epidemic, with a doubling time of approximately every six months. The initial cases of AIDS were concentrated in six metropolitan areas [*see Figure 2*].

Figure 2 **Reported cases of HIV/AIDS from June 1981 to September 1982.**

City	Cases	% of Total Cases
New York, NY	288	48.6
San Francisco, CA	78	13.2
Los Angeles, CA	37	6.2
Miami, FL	31	5.2
Newark, NJ	15	2.5
Houston, TX	15	2.5
Other	129	21.8
Total	593	100.0

This early study demonstrated the high frequency of AIDS cases in large metropolitan areas. New York, San Francisco, and Los Angeles were among the first cities in the U.S. to report cases of AIDS. These cities have remained at the forefront of the epidemic with regards to numbers of cases, complications, and new developments. But by now, cases are reported in almost all large and small cities in the United States, and across virtually all countries and continents on the globe. Worldwide, approximately 4000 people die of HIV/AIDS every day and this number is rapidly increasing.

THE ALARMS GO UNHEEDED

As the number of cases and deaths mounted in the early 1980s, a number of factors contributed to the lack of interest and funding to investigate the mounting epidemic. They were:

- homophobia,
- racism,
- prejudice, and
- puritanism.

In the United States and worldwide, HIV/AIDS has been erroneously labeled as a gay disease, when more than 80% of all cases across the globe are of heterosexual origins. In the past decade many groups in the U.S. have publicly condemned the gay population, going so far as to propose that the HIV/AIDS epidemic is God's punishment to gay men for their lifestyle. Obtaining funding for any issue related to the homosexual population was nearly impossible in the 1980's and remains very difficult today.

Racism is another factor. HIV/AIDS disproportionally attacks the African American population and the Hispanic population at a rate of two to five times that of Caucasian groups. Prejudice against non-whites as well as against those with HIV/AIDS has made it very difficult to fund research and social programs for these people.

And then there is our puritanism. Previously in the U.S., the discussion of sex and sexually transmitted diseases has been rigorously censored, and today it remains difficult. Even more than 15 years after the epidemic began in the U.S., HIV/AIDS education to elementary and high schools is very limited and public education on the disease is almost nonexistent. Condom ads and availability also remain scarce, and most people have no idea what "Safe Sex" practices involve.

THE LONG PERIOD BETWEEN INITIAL INFECTION AND SYMPTOMS

HIV confused many researchers by the long time period between initial infection with HIV and the onset of symptoms. For most viral infections, the time from infection to their most serious symptoms is two to four weeks. For HIV, the time from infection to serious disease ranges from two to 12 years. To connect an event in a person's life a decade earlier to his current fevers and multiple infections was something that had never been required before by any disease.

Additional factors that confused many physicians and researchers were the dizzying array of rare and lethal infections and cancers that occurred in people with HIV infection. Many physicians at first believed that the infections, Cytomegalovirus, or perhaps Pneumocystis carinii were the primary causes of the sickness and death of the first cases reported.

A further complication had to do with the system HIV attacked. The immune system is a complex array of cells and tissue covering and intertwined within the organs of the body. Its purpose is to protect us from infection and cancers, and if one occurs, to fight and get rid of it. The structure of the immune system was just beginning to be sorted in the mid 1970s. No one had imagined or seen an infection, much less a virus, that fed upon and devastated the very immune system cells that were supposed to be fighting it. In addition, the ability of this virus to change or mutate its appearance and function were unparalleled in medicine, and thwarted initial attempts to control or stop its destructive nature.

HIV IS DISCOVERED

In 1983 Dr. Luc Montagnier of the Pasteur Institute in France was the first to isolate the cause of the AIDS epidemic, a virus eventually named the Human Immunodeficiency Virus, or HIV. However, Dr. Montagnier and his team could only grow the virus for short periods of time in culture, because the virus destroyed the cells it grew in faster than technicians could replenish the culture. Dr. Robert Gallo followed Montagnier's work at the National Institutes of Health in Bethesda, Maryland and successfully grew and propagated HIV in culture, using a similar technique as Montagnier but with the addition of a T cell growth factor, Interleukin-2.

Once the virus was identified, an HIV test by antibody was developed, which allowed physicians and researchers worldwide to test well and sick patients to determine the extent of the epidemic.

THE WORLDWIDE SPREAD OF HIV/AIDS

Early French studies noted a significant association between early cases of AIDS and recent travel or immigration from Central Africa or the U.S. Many scientists now speculate that HIV has long infected isolated human populations in Central Africa, and only recently has spread in epidemic proportions due to the changes in social mobility and sexual attitudes in recent decades [*see Figure 3*]. Others suspect that HIV is the result of a more recent mutation of an animal retrovirus, enabling it to infect humans.

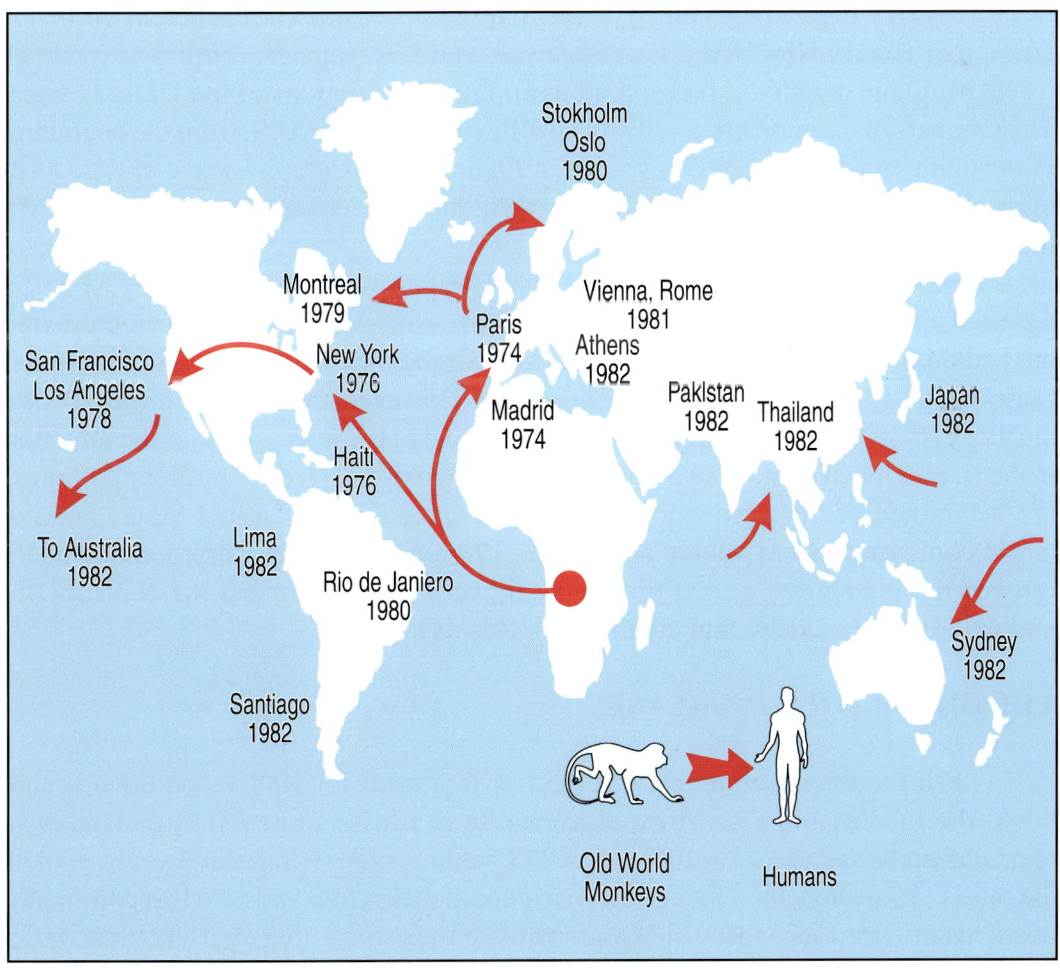

Figure 3 **The probable origin of HIV in Central Africa and its worldwide spread in the 1970's and 1980's (in red).**

It is likely that HIV originated in Central Africa sometime prior to 1960. The current epidemic gained momentum in the 1960s and spread rapidly in the 1970s. It probably expanded to other regions during the mid 1970s and 1980s, moving simultaneously to Europe and the United States, and later to Central and South America, Australia, and Asia. The probable dates of major transmission to the other regions of the world are indicated in *Figure 3* by the year overlying each region on the world map. These dates are calculated as two years prior to the first reported AIDS cases of the present epidemic in each region of the world.

THE NUMBER OF CASES OF HIV/AIDS MOUNTS

As HIV entered the United States, it quickly became entrenched in the major cities, particularly New York, San Francisco, and Los Angeles. Within 10 years of its entering this country, it had spread to all cities and regions of the United States. The numbers of cases of AIDS (advanced HIV disease) in the U.S. from the beginning of the epidemic through 1997 is shown in *Figure 4*. This graph has the classic form of an epidemic with a doubling time through the first decade of approximately six months to one year.

Since the Centers for Disease Control requires that only cases of AIDS be reported, the number of actual cases of HIV infection (with or without symptoms) in the United States can only be estimated. The number of cases of AIDS in the United States as of 1996 is 570,000 [*see Figure 4*]. However, this is only the tip of the iceberg. The estimated number of people infected by HIV at any stage of the infection in the U. S. is much higher and is currently estimated to be 1.0 to 1.7 million. Although the magnitude of this epidemic and its rapid spread in the United States and the world community were known as early as 1986, public and governmental leaders ignored the predictions at that time, and did very little to prevent the current U.S. and worldwide epidemic that continues to this day.

THE DEATH TOLL INCREASES

Prior to the development of effective treatment for HIV, as outlined in this book, the median life span from diagnosis to death for most AIDS patients was approximately one year. Virtually all AIDS patients died within three years of their diagnosis. Untreated, the cause of death in people with AIDS varies. Most commonly death results from secondary or "Opportunistic Infections" that overwhelm an HIV-weakened immune system to do deadly damage to the major organs of the body.

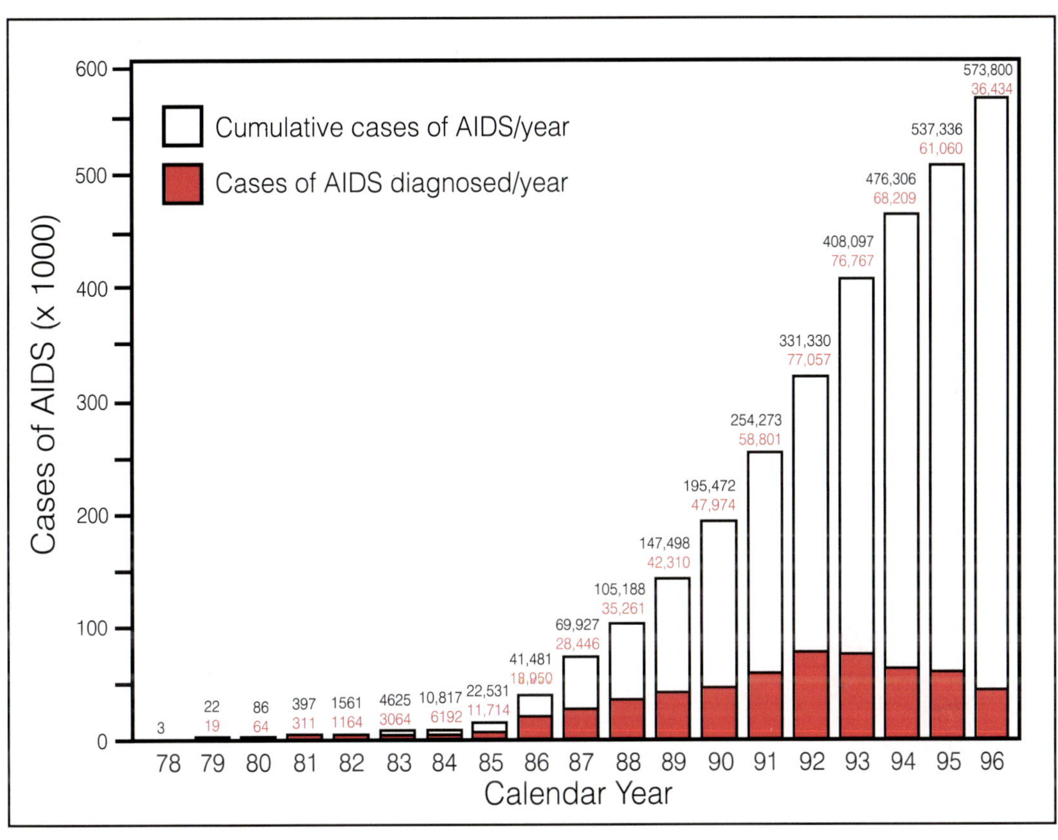

Figure 4 **The individual and cumulative number of AIDS cases in the U.S. from the years 1978 through 1996.**

The most common types of lethal infections in people with AIDS are protozoan, viral, and fungal infections. Pneumocystis carinii, Cryptococcus, Toxoplasma gondii, and Cryptosporidia are common fungal and protozoan infections. Pneumocystis carinii pneumonia (PCP), for example has an annual attack rate of approximately 35% to 70%, which is currently on the wane due to effective prevention medications, and public and physician education. Cytomegalovirus, or CMV, and other members of the Herpes virus family are common viral infections. The British sailor who may have been the first AIDS fatality in the West died of these same infections some 40 years ago. Bacterial infections are generally less of a problem. Malignancies or cancers, such as lymphomas, and Kaposi's Sarcoma (which is a viral sarcoma) also occur with increased frequency in people with HIV infection.

The number of deaths due to AIDS per year is approximately equal to the number of AIDS cases diagnosed in the previous year. *Figure 5* shows the cumulative deaths from HIV/AIDS in the United States from 1978 to the present. The disease is devastating men more than women, and African-American and Hispanic populations more than white populations. Estimates are that one in every three African-American men between the age of 21-45 years will die of AIDS.

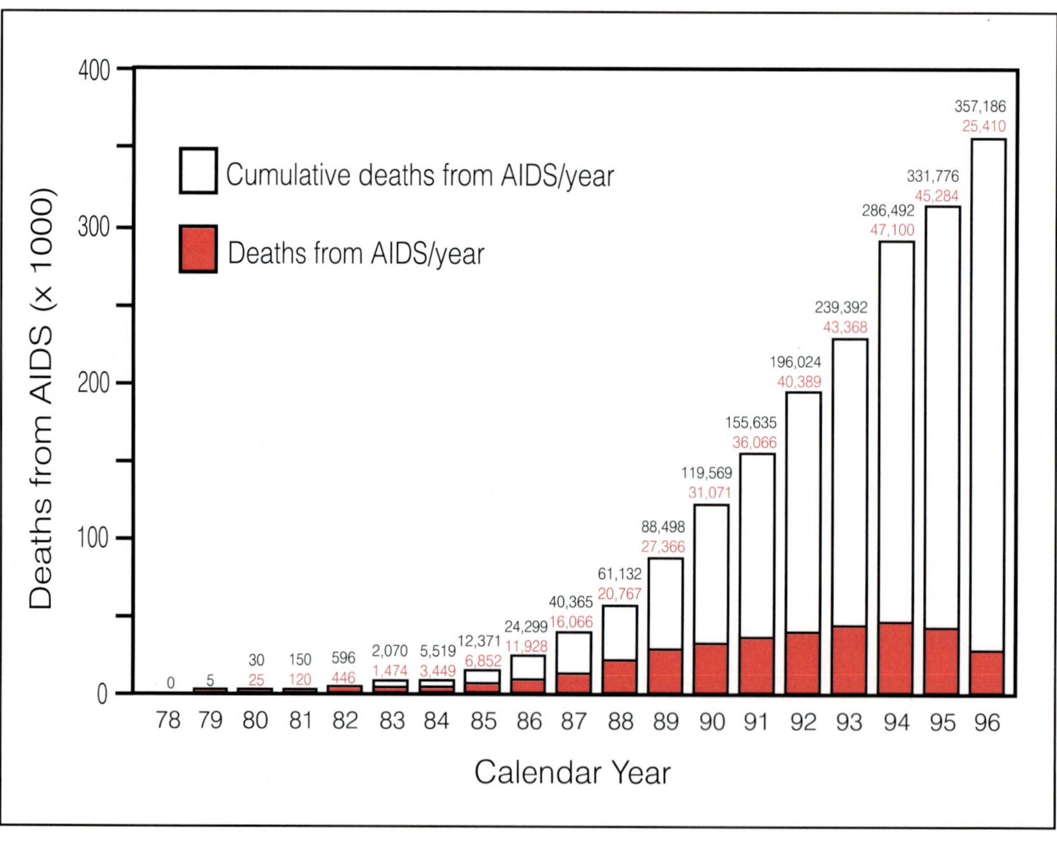

Figure 5 **The individual and cumulative number of deaths due to AIDS from 1978 through 1996.**

THE EPIDEMIC CONTINUES TO EXPAND

Worldwide the epidemic is still expanding rapidly. Each day an estimated 8500 people are newly infected. Of these 8500 new HIV cases:

- 1000 are children under the age of 15,
- 45 - 50% are females,
- 50% are young adults ages 15-25 years of age.

The numbers are daunting. In 1996, approximately 3.5 million new HIV infections occurred, 1.5 million people died of HIV/AIDS, and a total of 22.4 million people are now infected worldwide [*see Figure 6*].

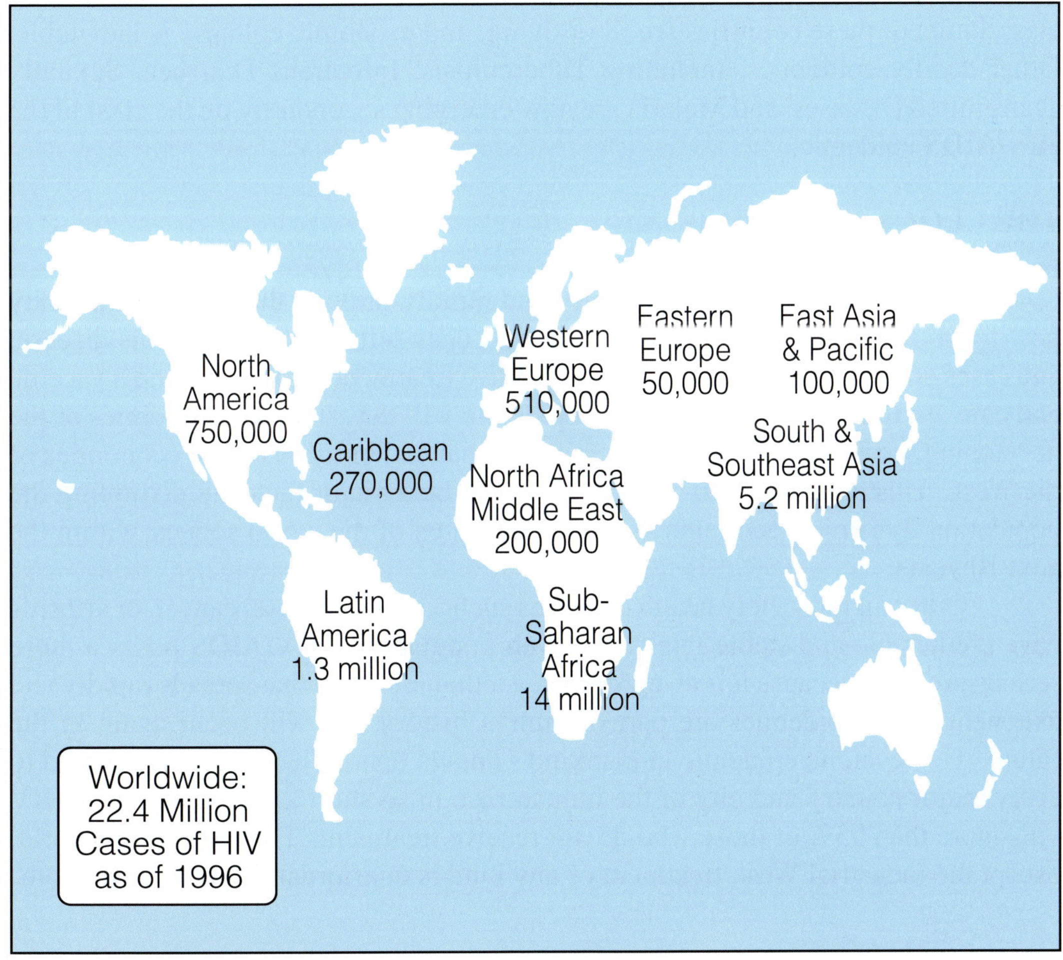

Figure 6 **The current distribution of HIV in the world community.**

Not unexpectedly, the greatest number of HIV/AIDS cases is in Central Africa, where the epidemic is most mature. However, South and Southeast Asia have just recently encountered HIV and already have a staggering 5.2 million cases. Their caseload is increasing exponentially, doubling every six to 12 months in many areas. We expect the Asian caseload to rapidly overtake and exceed the African epidemic within the next five years.

The devastation to the countries involved is almost unimaginable. In many African cities, more than 40% of pregnant women are infected with HIV, double the rate from two to three years ago. The average life span in many of these African countries has dropped by 10 years and continues to decline. Some countries don't expect any of their adults to live beyond the age of 40 or 45. In these places, 80% to 90% of hospital beds are occupied by people with HIV/AIDS, and there are not even the most rudimentary medicines to treat basic infections, much less HIV. The working class adults of these countries are ill or dying, and economic collapse is inevitable. Other deadly epidemics, including Tuberculosis, Infectious Diarrhea, Sexually Transmitted Diseases, and Malaria are now emerging secondarily on the crest of the HIV/AIDS epidemic.

THE CLOCK IS TICKING

HIV has been spreading silently and rapidly through the world community now for more than 20 years. No country has been left unaffected by this disease, and cases continue to increase. Unless effective treatment is provided and a vaccine and cure are found soon, this growing epidemic will devastate the economies of the developing world, and place ever increasing financial burdens on the economies of the West. Unstopped, the HIV epidemic could be a major factor in disrupting the population dynamics, economies, and social status of the world society within the next 10 years.

Other major society health concerns such as heart disease, cancer, or arthritis have predictable and stable rates in a given population. HIV/AIDS poses a more serious problem because it is an **epidemic**, a lethal infection that spreads rapidly and exponentially. Epidemics are part of human history and will occur again in the future. However, no epidemic in mankind's known history has so rapidly spread to every major country and city of the human race in so short a period of time. HIV kills more than 95% of those who do not receive treatment. For most of the world, except the industrial West, treatment of any kind is unaffordable and not available.

There is no more urgent medical need in the world today than stopping the HIV/AIDS epidemic. We **must** provide effective treatment and a cure for those infected, and an effective vaccine to prevent further spread of the.disease. It seems clear, therefore, that the world's resources should be allocated on an unlimited scale to producing the science and medical discoveries necessary to halt the HIV/AIDS epidemic. What we do now will determine the health and even the social strata of future generations worldwide.

2
HIV IS THE CAUSE

2 HIV IS THE CAUSE

HIV is an abbreviation for the **Human Immunodeficiency Virus**, the cause of AIDS and AIDS related illness. HIV is a life form called a virus. Within the family of viruses, it is known as a Retrovirus. HIV has had a number of different names, including: HTLV-III, or Human T-Cell Lymphotropic Virus, Type 3; LAV, or Lymphadenopathy Associated Virus; ARV, or AIDS Related Virus. In 1987, an international committee renamed the virus HIV to avoid the confusion of multiple names. With the isolation of different subtypes of this group of viruses, it is now designated as HIV-1. A slightly different form of the virus has been designated HIV-2.

TRANSMISSION OF HIV

The transmission of HIV, fortunately, is rather difficult compared to most viruses that infect mankind. HIV is transmitted almost exclusively through three modes of transmission, as listed below:

HIV is transmitted through sexual intercourse. By far, this is the major mode of transmission of HIV cases in the world. HIV is found heavily in semen and less so in mucous secretions.

HIV is transmitted from mother to child during pregnancy. The rate of transmission varies from 10% to 75% depending on the health of the mother, concurrent infections, nutrition, and the mode of delivery. In addition, a mother with HIV who breast feeds her newborn child runs a high risk of transmission of HIV to the child.

HIV is transmitted by injection using HIV contaminated needles or instruments. This is the usual mode of transmission for intravenous drug users. In addition, there have been a rare number of health care workers infected through accidental needle sticks, or injuries from contaminated scalpels or other sharp instruments. As in surgery, the risk of acquiring HIV infection in dentistry is not from a gloved, skilled dentist, but from unsterilized instruments that may have become contaminated with HIV from a previous patient. All surgical and dental instruments should be disposable or completely sterilized prior to use.

Like the rest of the world, the transmission of HIV in the United States has primarily been through unprotected sexual intercourse. But in Western Europe and the United States, it began within the gay or male homosexual population. As a result, in the U.S. and in Europe it is the male homosexual population who was hit first with the epidemic and continues to be hit the hardest. In contrast, in Central Africa where more than 60% of all worldwide HIV/AIDS cases occur, HIV infected the heterosexual population first, and as a result the vast majority of cases in Africa, and in the world, occur in the heterosexual populations.

WHAT IS A VIRUS?

The differences between viruses and other life forms are crucial to the understanding of their life cycle, the diseases they cause, and how we may combat them. A virus is among the smallest of life forms, measuring on average between 10 to 300 nm in diameter (nm=nanometer, which is .000000001 meter). In comparison to other objects, HIV is approximately 1000 times larger than an atom, and 10 to 100 times smaller than common bacteria. Viruses, by nature, are parasites because they are unable to replicate without infecting other life forms. Viruses can exist in an inactive state. Then they are inert matter and devoid of signs of life. When they encounter the appropriate host life form, they perform their only function in life, which is to replicate into new virus.

Viruses are unique in many ways from other higher order life forms:

- they are unable to function on their own,
- they require other organisms to replicate,
- they may be crystallized, where they behave as non-living matter,
- when they infect other organisms, they behave as living matter,
- they may lie dormant for long periods of time.

Although viruses are considered to be alive, they do not quite meet standard biology's definition of living matter. The seven properties of living matter are:

1. organization
2. reproduction
3. adaptation
4. metabolism
5. movement
6. irritability
7. growth

Viruses are organized structures, they reproduce, and they adapt to their environment through mutations (genetic changes) and natural selection during their replicative cycles. Thus, they meet three of the seven properties of living matter. However, they do not cycle energy on their own (metabolism), they do not move on their own (movement), they do not respond to stimuli (irritability), nor do they grow.

A VIRUS HAS A SIMPLE STRUCTURE

Viruses have a specific organization, which is a rather basic simple structure containing an outer layer of lipids (fats) and proteins surrounding genetic material of either DNA or RNA [*see Figure 1*].

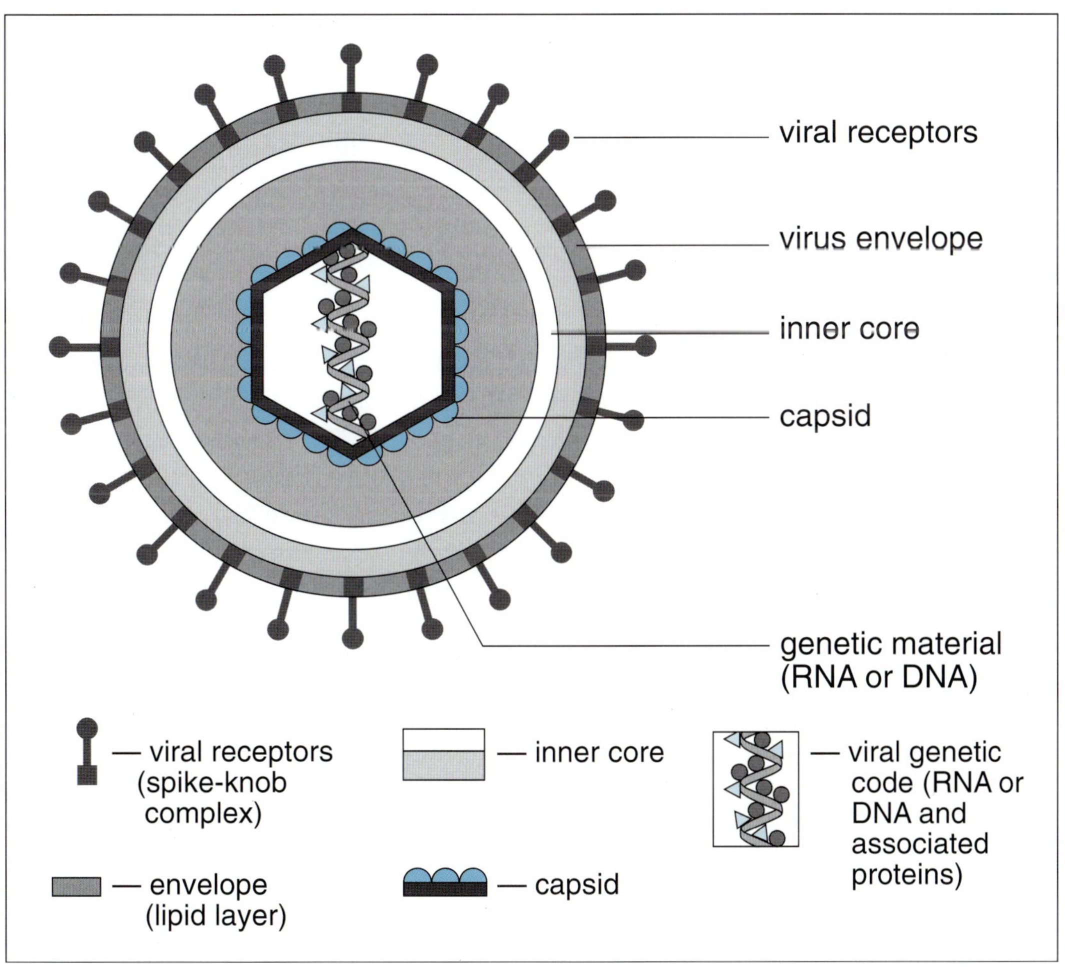

Figure 1 **Viruses are among the smallest and most simple of life forms.**

A virus has only one purpose: to transfer genetic material from itself into the cell or organism that it infects.

Most viruses have an outer coat or envelope, with receptors, whose purpose it is to bind to the host life form that they wish to infect. Frequently there is one or more inner layers of protein surrounding a central core structure. Within the core, which may also be called the capsid, is the genetic material that makes that particular virus unique from other viruses. Contained within the capsid are additional enzymes or substances that are crucial to the viral replication cycle, such as ribonuclease, protease, reverse transcriptase, and integrase, depending on the type and family of the virus.

Viruses belong to the Kingdom of life forms called Prokarya, which also includes other simple life forms such as bacteria and blue-green algae. Among the Viruses, HIV is in the Family: Retroviridae, Subfamily: Lentivirinae, and Genus: Lentivirus. Other members of this subfamily include the Simian Immunodeficiency Virus (SIV in monkeys), the Visna Virus (sheep), the Caprine Arthritis Encephalitis Virus (goats), and the Equine Infectious Anemia Virus (horses). These viruses cause chronic inflammatory disease in their hosts.

HIV IS A RETROVIRUS

The Retroviridae, more commonly referred to as Retroviruses, are a newly discovered family of viruses first described in the 1970s. They are different from all other viruses in a very unique way. Most viruses and, for that matter, most life forms replicate in a forward direction, going from DNA to RNA to protein, or simply from RNA to protein. The Retroviruses like HIV and its cousins replicate in a backward or "retro" direction from RNA to DNA, then from DNA to RNA, then from RNA to protein [*see Figure 2*]. This unusual backward stepping is made possible by a unique chemical called reverse transcriptase, or "RT" for short.

What is the purpose of this unusual step of retro-replication? And why would a virus evolve backward rather than forward? HIV and other retroviruses do it to survive. By moving into a DNA form, the virus appears similar to one's own human genetic code. Then HIV uses a unique chemical, called integrase, to integrate or "cut open" and insert itself into human genes, where it can effectively "hide" from the human immune defenses to emerge at will when the environment is suitable. The result of allowing retroviral DNA to be integrated into the human genes is the difficult and chronic lifelong infections that the Retroviruses, including HIV, are known for.

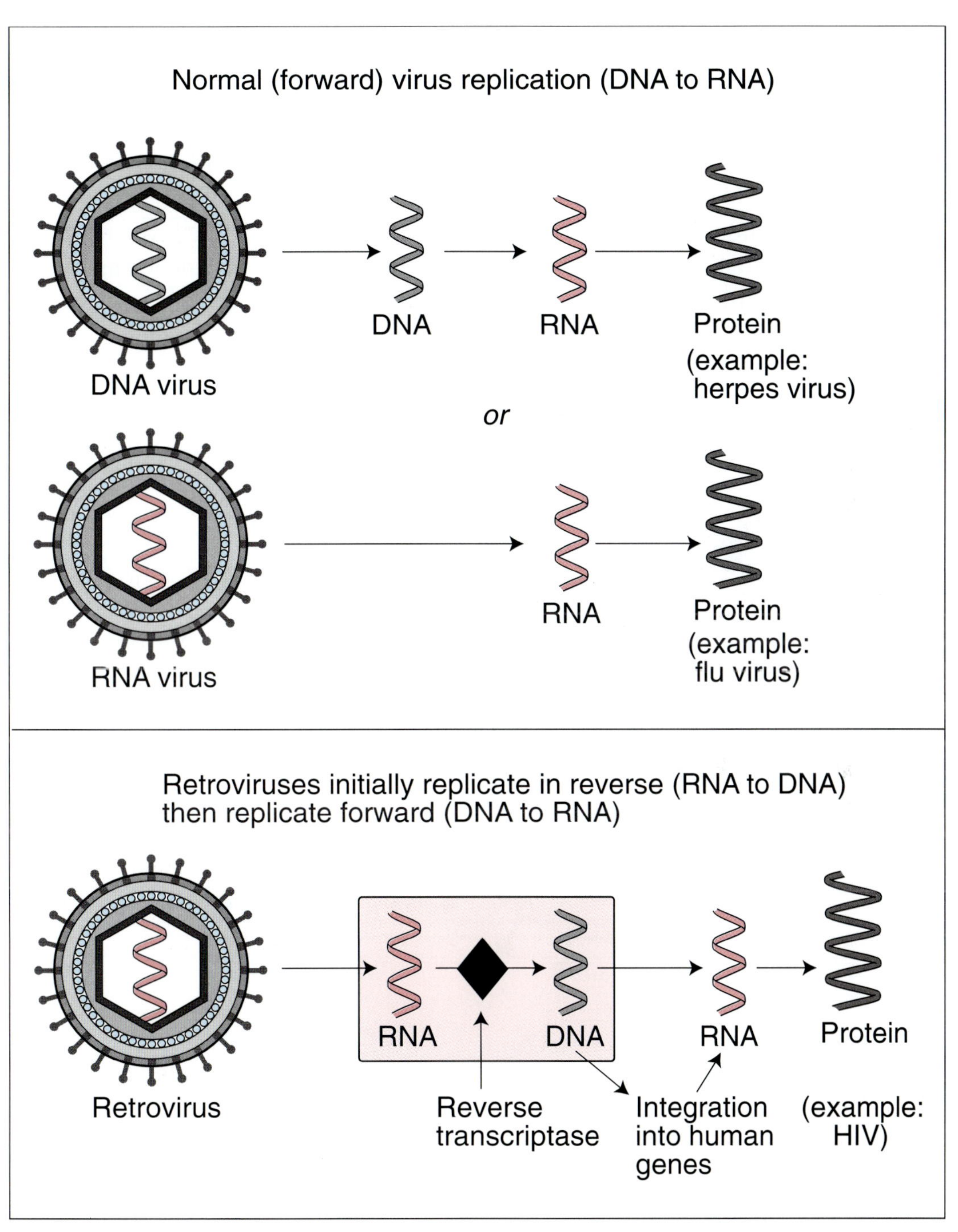

Figure 2 **Retroviruses (HIV) replicate initially in a reverse or "retro" direction compared to common viruses (like Herpes, flu viruses).**

HIV VIRAL STRUCTURE

HIV is a medium sized virus. It has an outer surface made of lipid [fat] that contains spike-knob projections called gp120 receptors [*see Figure 3*]. These receptors bind HIV to the receptors of the cells that HIV attacks. The HIV gp120 receptors are anchored to the outer membrane of HIV by a particular protein referred to as gp41. The combination of the HIV receptor gp120 and its anchoring protein gp41, forms a third protein, gp160, all of which will turn up on any positive HIV antibody test.

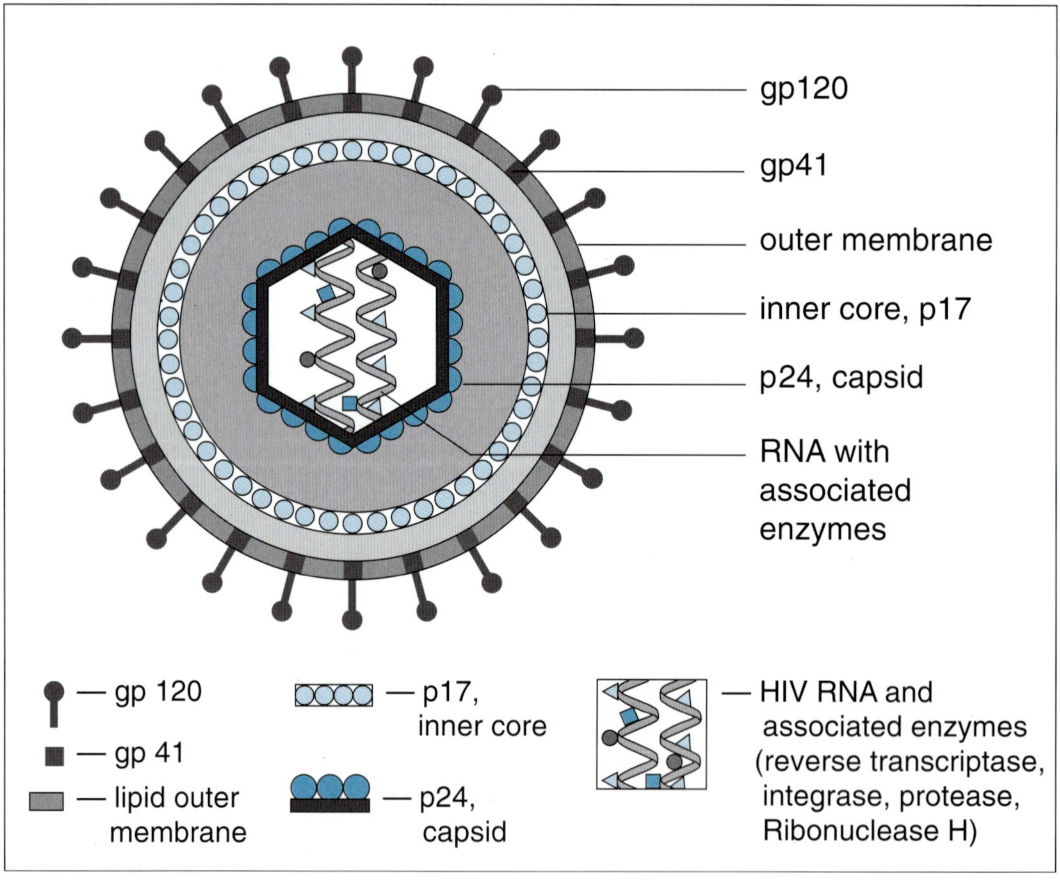

Figure 3 **The structure of HIV includes outer receptors of glycoprotein 120 (gp120) and gp41, an inner layer of protein 17 (p17), and a capsid made up of p24, containing two strands of RNA.**

The inner core layer (p17) probably stabilizes the structure of the virus. Below the inner core lies the capsid (p24) which carries the genetic coding data of HIV RNA and key enzymes needed to initiate and complete HIV replication. These enzymes include reverse transcriptase, integrase, ribonucleaseH, and protease. Reverse transcriptase (RT) acts in the early phase of HIV replication, actually performing the "retro" step, converting HIV RNA into HIV DNA. Integrase works in mid phase HIV replication, by cutting and inserting the newly formed HIV DNA into the human DNA genetic code. RibonucleaseH assists in the production of HIV double-stranded DNA. HIV protease functions in late phase HIV replication by processing and converting the newly formed HIV viruses from non-infectious particles to mature infectious HIV.

HIV REPLICATION

The HIV genetic code is about one-tenth the size of the genetic code of other viruses, and is simple, containing only nine sections, called genes [*see Figure 4*]. The genetic code is basically instructions to replicate the new virus that fuels the ongoing infection in each person with HIV. The genes *gag, pol,* and *env* produce proteins that form the core, enzymes, and envelope of the new HIV particles. *Vif, vpr, vpu, tat, rev,* and *nev* regulate this process. The most important of these is the *tat* gene which regulates the replication rate of HIV, one of the fastest replicating human viruses yet discovered.

The replication cycle of HIV can be divided into three phases, which consist of ten steps. To understand how we attack HIV, one should be familiar with the ten basic steps of HIV replication shown in *Figure 5* and described below:

1. **cell binding**
2. **penetration**
3. **uncoating**
4. **reverse transcription**
5. **nuclear integration**
6. **transcription**
7. **translation**
8. **assembly**
9. **budding**
10. **maturation (protease)**

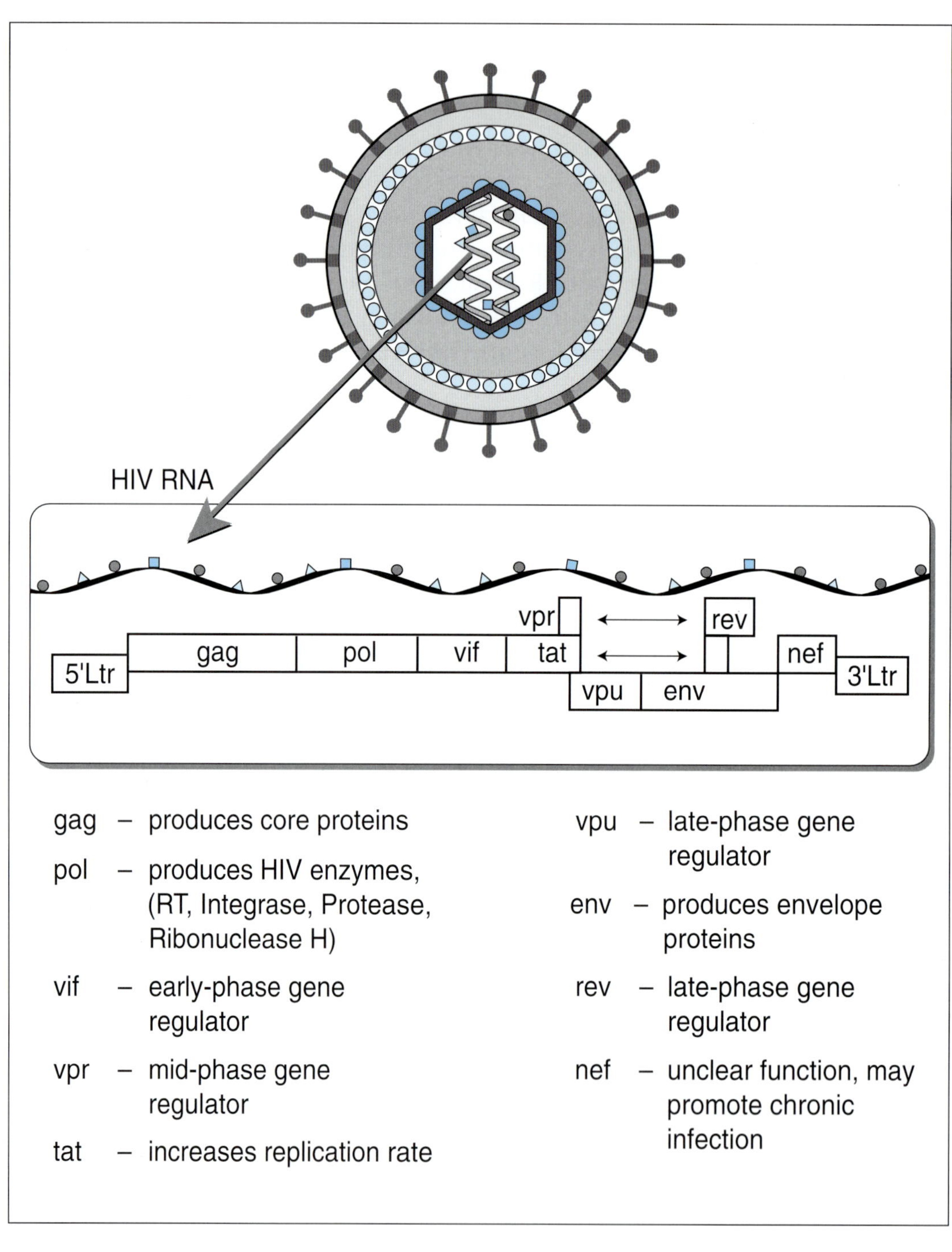

Figure 4 **The nine genes of the HIV genetic code, RNA.**

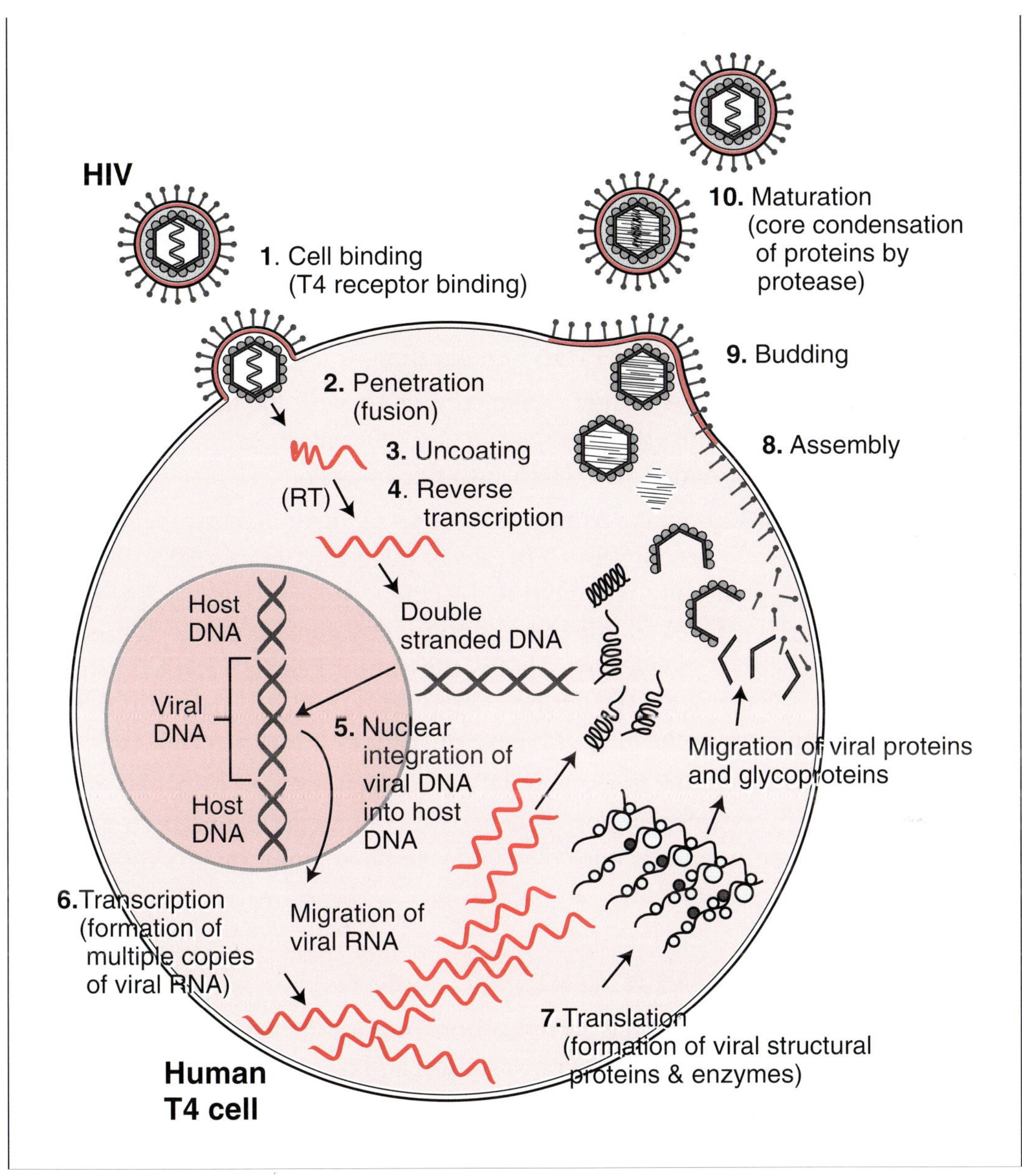

Figure 5 **The HIV replication cycle contains ten steps.**

EARLY PHASE REPLICATION: cell binding, penetration, uncoating, and reverse transcription

1. Cell binding is the binding of HIV gp 120 receptors to the T4 cell receptors. At least 90% of the cells HIV infects are T4 cells and the remaining 10% include macrophages, dendritic cells, and microglial cells.

2. Penetration is the merger of HIV with the T4 cell membrane.

3. Uncoating occurs as T4 cell chemicals dissolve the HIV viral capsid, releasing strands of HIV RNA into the T4 cell.

4. Reverse transcription is the conversion of HIV RNA to HIV DNA through the actions of two viral enzymes: reverse transcriptase and ribonucleaseH. Reverse transcriptase creates HIV DNA from HIV RNA as it moves down the RNA. At the same time ribonucleaseH assists by dissolving the HIV RNA, as it is no longer needed.

MID PHASE REPLICATION: integration, transcription, and translation

5. Integration is the merger of the HIV DNA with the human genes of the T4 cell. In this step the enzyme integrase acts to cut and insert or "integrate" the newly formed double stranded HIV DNA into the T4 gene.

6. Transcription occurs as new HIV RNA is made (transcribed) from the integrated HIV DNA. When HIV DNA begins to manufacture new HIV depends on a number of factors, including whether the T4 cell is in an active or passive mode, the site where the HIV DNA is integrated into the T4 gene, and the characteristic genetic pattern of the HIV of that case. Half of the transcribed HIV RNA is processed to form the RNA for the new HIV virions being produced, and half of it serves as RNA for the production of the gag, pol, env, and other viral gene products.

7. Translation occurs as the new HIV RNA is translated from genetic RNA code to large protein complexes (polyproteins). As unprocessed polyproteins, these molecules are not yet functional until they undergo the maturation process provided by HIV protease.

LATE PHASE REPLICATION: assembly, budding and maturation

8. Assembly involves the complex construction of new HIV virions from the HIV products that resulted from transcription and translation.

9. Budding follows assembly. In budding, the new HIV pushes its way through the cell membrane, taking a piece of the membrane with it, which forms the outer coat.

10. Maturation is the final step in HIV replication. Although the new HIV virions have now floated away from the T4 cell where they were made, they are still in an immature, non-infectious form. HIV protease proceeds to process the large polyproteins of these new HIV virions, cutting them into shorter mature proteins. After this final step the new HIV virions are now infectious and float away looking for new T4 cells to start the replication process over again.

HIV REPLICATION DYNAMICS

The entire HIV replication cycle takes approximately two days. Each infected T4 cell produces about 100 new HIV virions per cell (a virion is a newly produced HIV virus). In an untreated person, there are approximately 10 billion new HIV virions produced each day [see Figure 6].

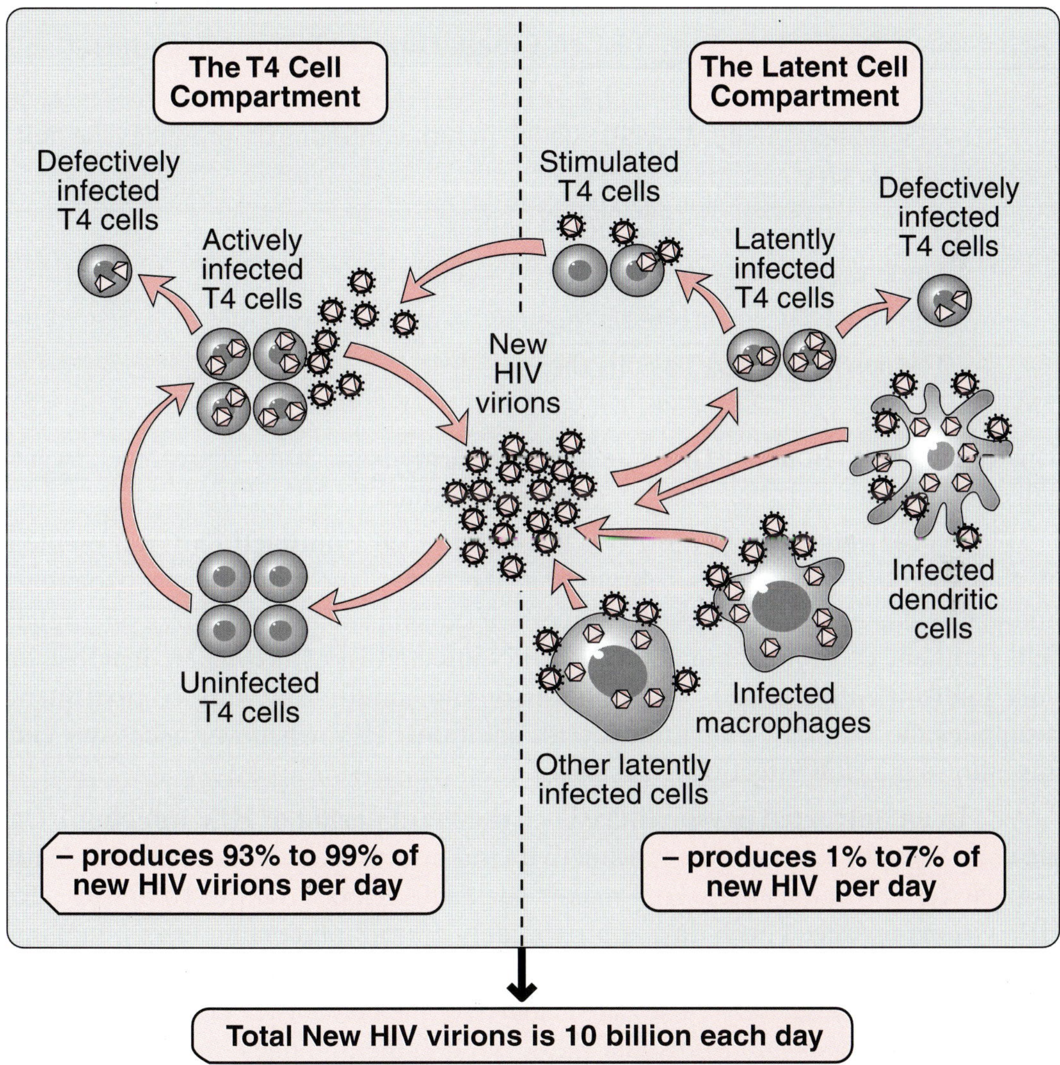

Figure 6 **The two "compartments" of HIV replication in the human body: the T4 Cell Compartment where most HIV is made, and the Latent Cell Compartment which "refuels" the HIV infection and maintains chronic infection.**

- **93% to 99%** of new HIV (virions) are produced from actively infected T4 cells, henceforth known as the **T4 Cell Compartment**, and

- **1% to 7%** come from latently (slow producing) infected cells, such as macrophages, latent T4 cells, microglial cells, and dendritic cells, henceforth known as the **Latent Cell Compartment**.

On the left of the diagram is the **T4 Cell Compartment**. In this compartment,

- HIV rapidly infects T4 cells, which in turn continuously produces the bulk of new HIV.
- In the process, these infected T4 cells die.
- The body attempts to make more T4 cells.
- The new HIV virions infect the new T4 cells.
- The newly infected T4 cells die.

This is the "battle front" of HIV infection: one army is the body, represented by T4 cells, and the enemy is the viral infection, represented by HIV virions.

On the right side of *Figure 6* is the **Latent Cell Compartment**, represented by a diverse cell group spread throughout the body: the macrophages (roaming immune cells), the dendritic cells (relay cells of the skin and lymph tissue), microglial cells (immune cells of the brain), and latently infected T4 cells (that are inactive, or only intermittently active). Continuously and indefinitely, this compartment resupplies the T4 Cell Compartment with additional HIV whenever necessary and thus allows the HIV infection to go on for years.

In an untreated person there is no dormant period of HIV infection. On the contrary, HIV is one of the most active viral infections ever encountered. With its massive replication cycle, HIV makes constant "errors." Of the 10 billion new HIV virions produced each day, approximately 10 million contain errors, making them different than those produced the day before. These changed HIV virions are called mutants or mutations. They are a source of the diversity of HIV, and account for why HIV evolves into forms that break through the immune defenses and form resistance to medicines when one takes a "soft approach" to treatment.

A "soft approach" is any treatment that only partially shuts down HIV replication. If HIV is able to replicate at all, it produces mutations that eventually break through treatment. **It is only when aggressive therapy is applied that completely and continuously blocks all HIV replication, that HIV ceases to evolve or mutate.**

SINGLE, DOUBLE, & TRIPLE THERAPY

Mathematical modeling of the HIV replication cycle shows that single therapy resistance occurs as rapidly as in one to 30 days and predictably will always fail to help a person with HIV infection. Single therapy is defined as the treatment of HIV infection with only one medication. Double or combination therapy, defined as treatment using two simultaneous medications, may develop resistance within three to six months. Furthermore, when it fails, combination therapy has actually succeeded in producing an HIV strain in its host that is resistant to both of the medications used in the combination.

Theoretically, triple therapy, defined as treatment using three effective medicines simultaneously, should prevent resistance for an estimated 10,000 years of treatment. This figure is based on a well-tested mathematical model of HIV replication that includes its replication rate, its mutation rate, and the time it would take for the virus to produce a mutant HIV strain with three simultaneous specific errors (mutations). Whether it's 100 years, 1000 years, or 10,000 years is not that important. The point is that it would take a very long time. But for the therapy to work, all three medicines must be taken continuously, according to directions, and all three medicines must be individually effective in that case at the onset of therapy.

The initiation of triple therapy has taught us some very useful things. We've learned that HIV is quickly shut down and rapidly cleared from the body of an infected person in two phases after effective triple therapy is begun, vacating the T4 Cell Compartment rapidly over 1-14 days, and clearing from the Latent Cell Compartment more slowly over one to two years, depending on the extent of the infection [*see Figure 7*].

Effective triple therapy not only shuts off HIV infection, but is able to clear about 95% of all HIV infection from the body, including the lymph nodes, thymus, blood, and central nervous system of an infected person within one to two years of treatment. All that remains is a small amount of HIV proviral DNA in the human chromosomes (genes) which we do not yet know how to clear. Our "cure projects" will now be directed at finding ways to eliminate this remaining 5% of HIV infection from a treated person. Until we find that solution, triple therapy will have to be continued diligently, because as soon as a person stops taking his medications, those 5% of HIV remaining will reactivate and begin spreading and reseeding the lymph nodes, thymus, blood, and other parts of the body.

It is not surprising that the increase in T4 cell count, demonstrating the improved health of the immune system, appears to improve in two phases, in response to the two phase reduction of HIV with effective triple therapy [*see Figure 8*].

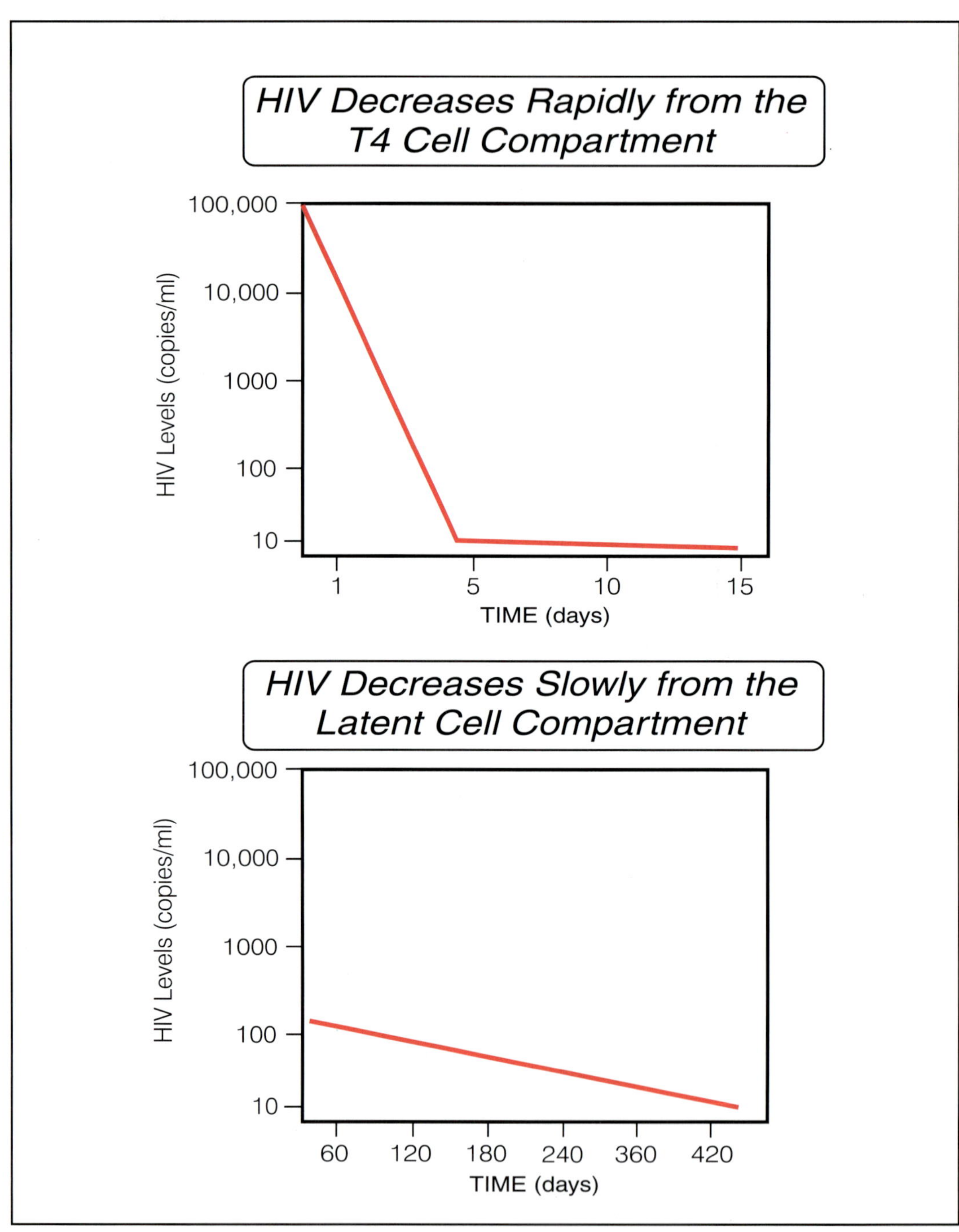

Figure 7 **The level of HIV infection decreases with triple therapy. More than 90% of HIV is shut off quickly in the T4 Cell Compartment by day 14. HIV in the Latent Cell Compartment is more difficult to shut off and takes more than one year.**

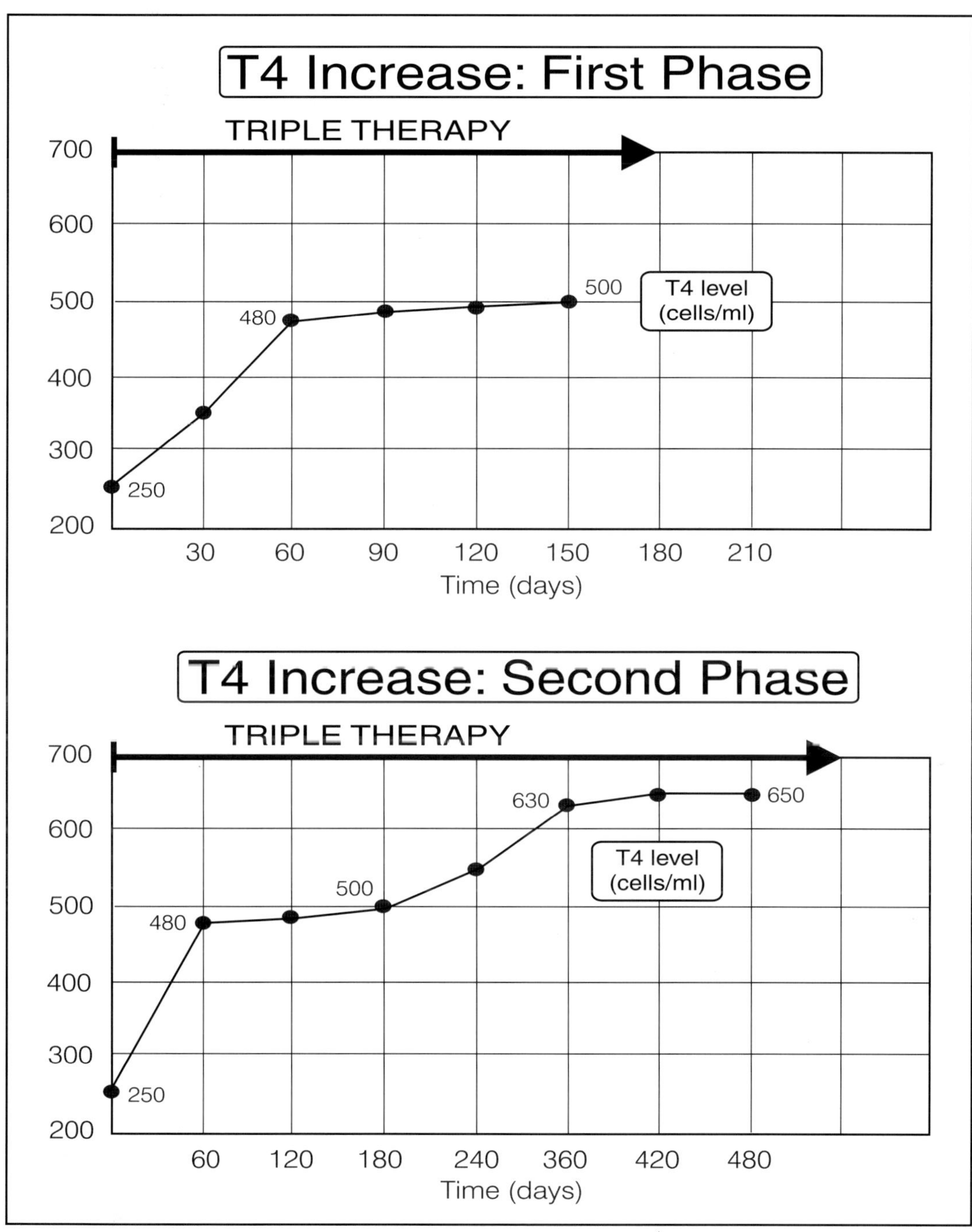

Figure 8 **The immune system as measured by a rising T4 cell count improves as HIV infection is shut off by triple therapy. The initial improvement occurs in the first one to three months, and the second improvement occurs much later.**

The initial increase in T4 count occurs between days 30 to 60 and stabilizes at a higher level some months after, in response to the rapid clearance of HIV from the T4 Cell Compartment. The second increase in T4 count occurs about one year later in response to the gradual clearance of HIV from the Latent Cell Compartment. With one minor difference, the T4 count increases in direct response to the elimination of HIV infection. The increase in T4 count is typically delayed by 30 to 60 days from the drop in HIV level. It is likely this delay is the time the immune system takes to begin repairs once HIV infection is reduced.

Mathematical modeling and actual patient studies now confirm that:

- **HIV is highly active at all times**, producing more than 10 billion new HIV virions per day in an untreated HIV infected person,

- **single therapy is useless,**

- **double (combination) therapy is of limited use** and leads to multi-resistant HIV strains that respond poorly to therapy,

- **triple therapy shuts HIV off in two phases** (if all three medications are effective at one time),

- **the immune system improves in two phases**, as measured by T4 response after beginning effective triple therapy,

- **triple therapy, when properly applied, clears 90% to 95% of HIV from the body of an infected person,** and

- **triple therapy, when properly applied, should have an extremely long, and possibly indefinite benefit to those taking the therapy.**

3
THE COURSE OF HIV INFECTION
Without Treatment

3 THE COURSE OF HIV INFECTION

Without Treatment

HIV infects and kills immune system cells in the body, primarily T4 cells, although it may also infect other cells of the immune system, such as macrophages, dendritic cells, and microglial cells [*see Figure 1*].

When we say HIV "infects" T4 cells, we mean that HIV enters the T4 cell and replicates into hundreds of new HIV particles, a process that kills the T4 cells. The time from infection of a T4 cell to the production of new HIV virions is about two days. Billions of new HIV particles are produced each day in an infected person who does not take therapy to stop HIV replication.

HIV also infects macrophage cells that migrate throughout the body as part of their immune system function. Infected macrophages are nonfunctional, and produce new HIV particles slowly over a number of weeks or longer. Infected macrophages are a chronic reservoir for HIV because these cells may live for weeks or even months before dying.

The immune system relay cell, the dendritic cell, is also chronically infected by HIV. Dendritic cells exist throughout the immune system, with major groups in the lymph nodes, skin, and gastrointestinal tract. This cell is another major reservoir of HIV and plays a key role in maintaining chronic HIV infection. As circulating T4 cells link with the dendritic relay cells, HIV is passed from the dendritic cells to the T4 cell population. As a higher percentage of the immune system dendritic population is infected, more and more T4 cells are infected and then rapidly killed by HIV. Meanwhile, the infected dendritic cells die slowly, forming scar tissue, an eerie tracing of the systematic destruction of the structure of the immune system.

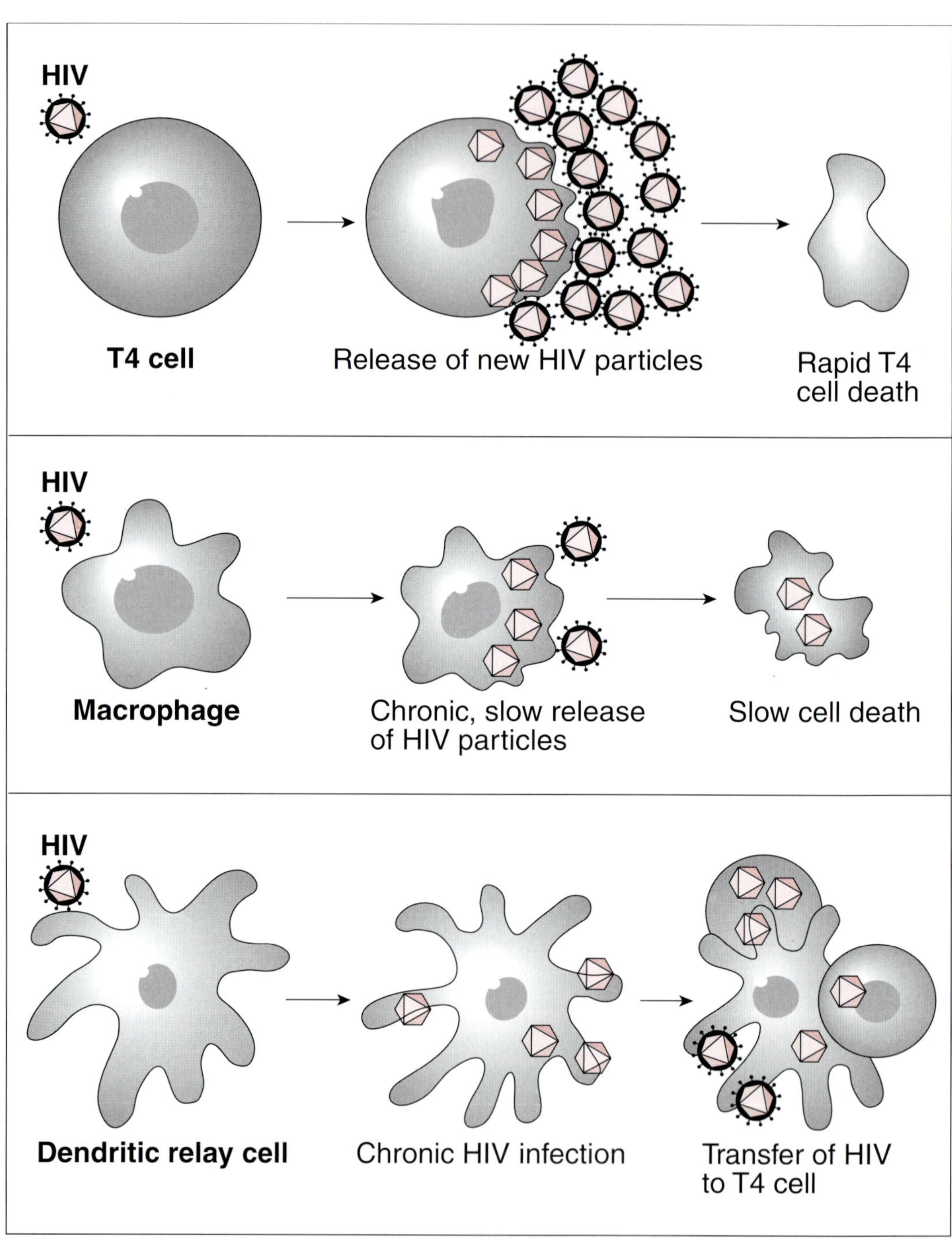

Figure 1 **HIV infects three major cell lines of the immune system: the T4 cell, the macrophage, and the dendritic cell, causing cell dysfunction followed by cell death.**

THE STRUCTURE OF THE HUMAN IMMUNE SYSTEM

Humans, as well as all species of animals, are awash in potentially infectious agents, including bacteria, virus, fungus, and various protozoa. A simple culture or scraping of any part of the skin or gastrointestinal tract from mouth to anus grows a plethora of organisms. We call this "normal flora." However, a culture of blood or any **internal** tissue of a healthy person reveals absolutely no such agents—no organisms at all other than that person's own cells.

How is this sterile internal environment maintained? This is the venue of the immune system, operating through a system of migrating cells, proteins, nodal tissue, and tissue covering [*see Figure 2*]. Without an immune system, death is very rapid.

Skin, and the linings of our gastrointestinal and respiratory tracts provide the barriers between the outside world of potentially infectious organisms and the sterile internal environment. Lymph nodes, the immune system gland called the thymus, and the lymphatic vessels form a system of relay tissue through which circulates a large volume of clear lymphatic fluid. This system of nodes, vessels and lymphatic fluid allows the immune system cells, such as the T cells and macrophages to migrate throughout the body. The critical dendritic relay cells live within the lymph nodes, skin, and gastrointestinal and respiratory linings.

HIV DESTROYS THE STRUCTURE OF THE IMMUNE SYSTEM

We have described the cellular damage of HIV on the T4 cell population, on macrophages, and on dendritic cells. There have also been numerous studies on the effects of HIV infection on the structure of the immune system. When HIV infects the lymph nodes of the immune system, the nodes expand, both internally and externally, in an attempt to trap and fight the HIV infection. These enlarged or "hyperplastic" lymph nodes are found on exam in most people within four weeks of HIV infection. Thus affected, lymph node tissue will show loss of T4 cells, increases in supportive immune cells, known as T8 cells, and a disorganized pattern of the dendritic and macrophage cell lines.

With time, HIV causes severe scarring of the lymph node structure which results in lymph node shrinkage, called atrophy [*see Figure 2, insert*]. Ultimately, the lymph system will demonstrate an absence of T4 cells, and an almost complete loss of other cell lines of the lymph nodes, including T8, dendritic cells, and the macrophage cell lines. In the final atrophied state, the immune system is in a state of collapse, unable to make T4 cells at all and unable to control HIV infection.

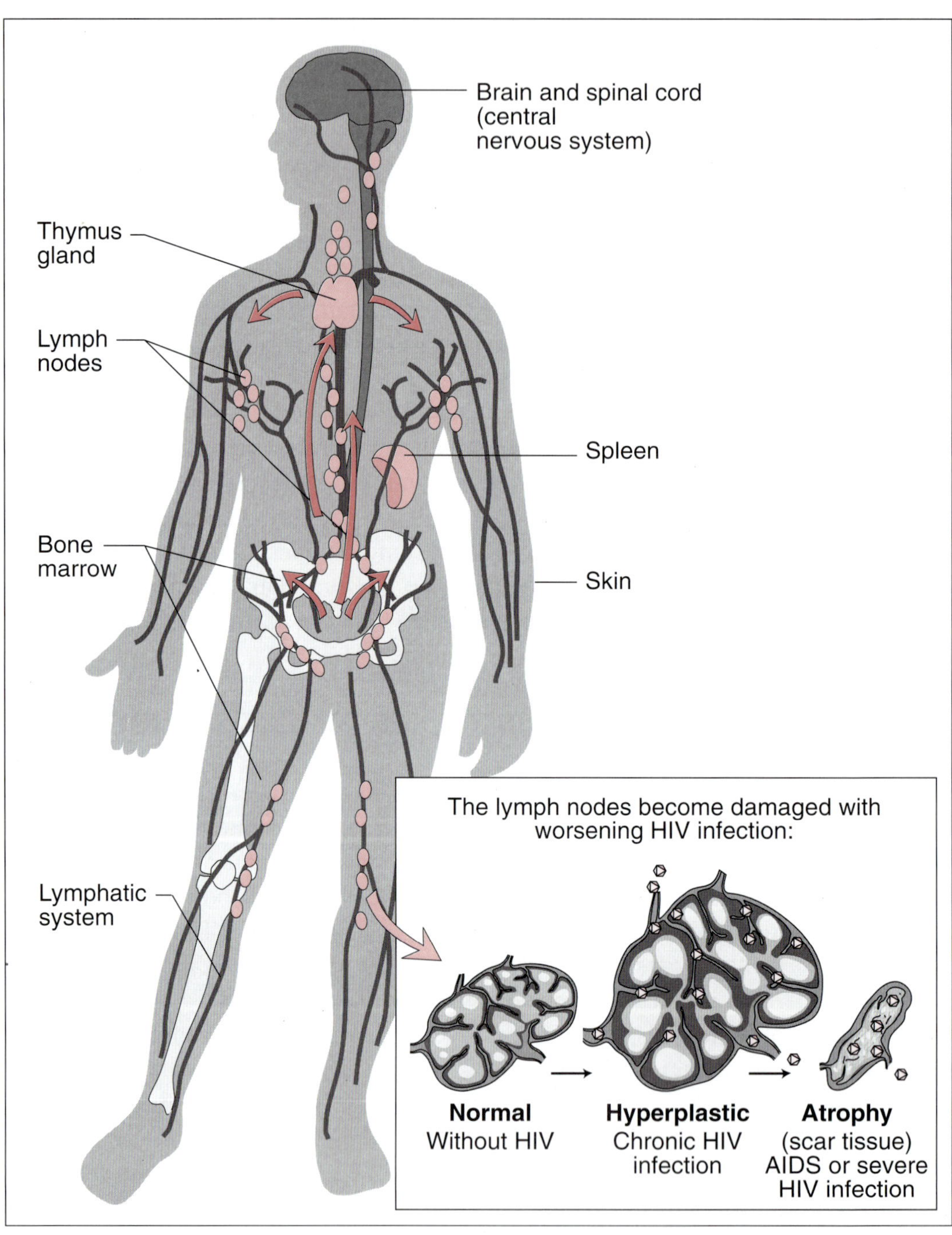

Figure 2 **The human immune system consists of its central organ, the thymus gland, and a network of tissue including the lymph nodes, lymphatic system, spleen, bone marrow, and skin. The lymph nodes become damaged and eventually nonfunctional as HIV infection worsens [*insert*].**

In this final state, people with HIV have AIDS, a severe lack of T4 cells with exceedingly high HIV viral levels and an extreme vulnerability to multiple, lethal infections and cancers. This condition of lymph node scarring is also called "lymph node burn out." Other parts of the immune system, including skin, mucous membranes, spleen, and thymus gland will demonstrate similar devastation by HIV. With the body's internal system decimated, and its external coverings severely damaged, it is not surprising that in Advanced HIV infection we find:

- a lack of palpable lymph nodes,

- frequent skin infections,

- frequent, chronic mouth and intestinal ulcers,

- frequent sinus and lung infections,

- potentially lethal internal infections consisting primarily of viral, fungal, protozoan, and encapsulated bacterial infections, and

- poor response to medical therapies that would normally cure a healthy person of these infections.

THE NATURAL, UNTREATED COURSE OF HIV INFECTION

The "natural course of infection" is how a disease evolves if no treatment is attempted to halt it. There are volumes of data on the natural course of HIV infection, as the epidemic was almost 10 years old and 100,000 were dead before combination therapy became available in 1990 to slow the disease. Unfortunately the medical establishment continued to recommend no therapy or ineffective single therapy with AZT until 1996. The reasons for this are not clear, but are probably due to a lack of national leadership at the time, bureaucratic delays, and a sense of hopelessness and caution due to previous treatment failures. It wasn't until 1996, with volumes more data on HIV disease, and an additional 250,000 more dead of it in the United States that effective treatment, in the form of combination and triple therapy, was formally endorsed by the HIV medical establishment.

Fifteen years of data on this disease tells us that untreated, HIV infection progresses through three stages: **Acute, Chronic**, and **Advanced (AIDS)**. The duration of each stage varies from case to case depending on one's health, one's genetics, the virulence of the particular HIV strain, and possibly the dose of the initial infection. Note that **these timelines are based on no treatment.** With effective treatment, people with HIV should not get AIDS. **Untreated**, the duration of each stage on average is:

Stage 1 (Acute HIV infection): one to three months,

Stage 2 (Chronic HIV infection): two to 10 years,

Stage 3 (Advanced HIV infection, AIDS): six months to two years.

Figure 3 graphs the T4 cell count over the three stages of HIV infection based on studies of individuals who did not receive HIV therapy for their conditions.

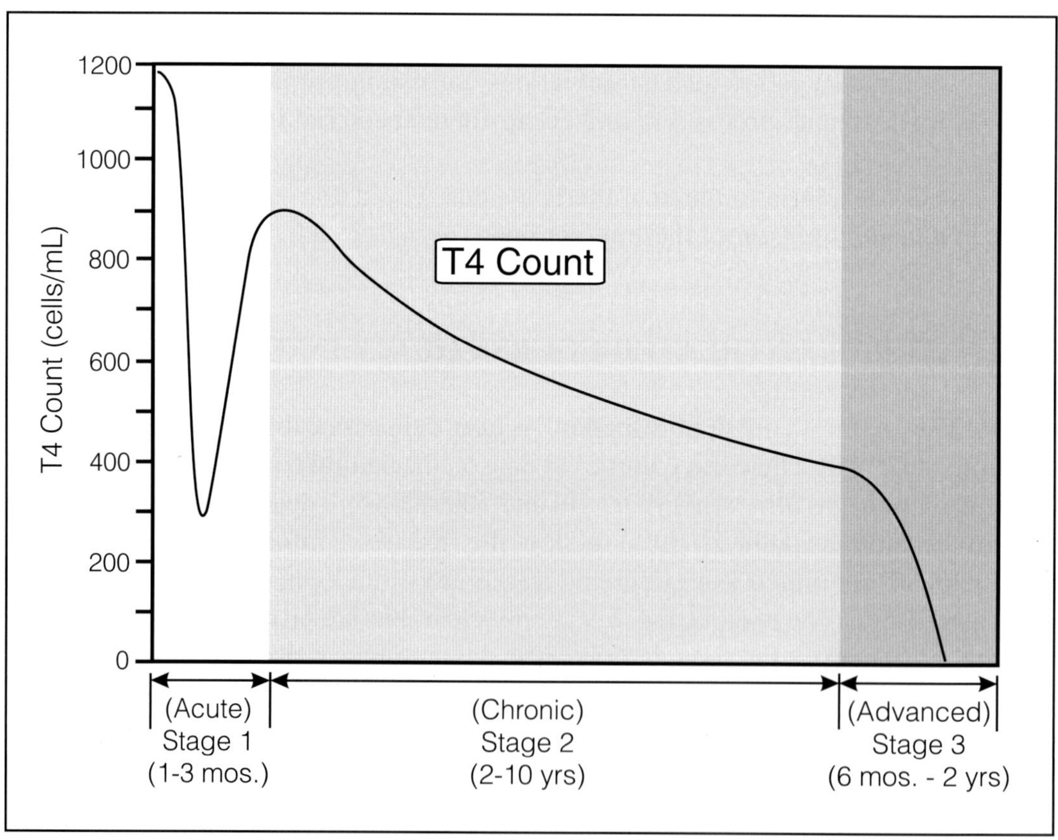

Figure 3 **The T4 count initially falls then recovers during Acute HIV, slowly declines during Chronic HIV, and rapidly declines to zero during Advanced HIV.**

During Stage 1, the T4 count abruptly drops from a level above 1000 to approximately 200, but recovers. During Stage 2, while HIV is replicating relentlessly throughout the immune system, there's a gradual fall in the T4 count that averages a loss of about 75 points per year. In Stage 3, the T4 count declines further as the remainder of the immune system fails. One is now vulnerable to many lethal infections and cancers.

In the beginning, in the early 1980s, it was thought that only a small proportion of those infected with HIV would die. By the mid 1980s, my research and that of my colleagues at San Francisco General Hospital demonstrated that at least 75% of those infected would progress to Stage 3 disease and die. We now know that more than 95% of those with HIV infection will die unless treatment is undertaken to stop the disease.

STAGE 1: ACUTE HIV INFECTION

Within two to three weeks of initial infection with HIV, one typically becomes acutely ill. Less often, these early symptoms are mild. The most common symptoms with the percentage reported in a large series of Stage 1 infections are:

Severe tiredness/malaise	89%
Fever/sweats	84%
Muscle/joint aches	84%
Sore throat	77%
Enlarged lymph nodes	71%
Headaches/light sensitivity	68%
Nausea/vomiting/appetite loss	58%
Diffuse body rash	53%
Diarrhea	32%

A person might think he had a bad case of the flu. Fevers are typically 101 to 102 degrees Fahrenheit, but may be as high as 106. Sometimes this Acute stage looks like a common upper respiratory "cold," except that it lasts from four to 12 weeks, is more intense than a cold, and includes other diffuse symptoms. Rarely, some patients in this stage progress to meningeal signs (severe headache and confusion) and coma.

Laboratory data in Stage 1 is unremarkable except for a shift towards production of virus-fighting white cells, called lymphocytes. A mild elevation of the liver function tests may occur, usually without clinical symptoms. The illness usually runs its course without serious events, except dehydration, and some mild discomfort. As the immune system returns to normal, and the symptoms are receding, the infected person may break out in a diffuse body rash. The rash produces no symptoms, occurs in more than 50% of cases and disappears without treatment within two weeks of its appearance. This rash is called a "viral exanthem," a common immune complex rash seen in many viral illness as they are resolving.

After HIV enters the body, it rapidly spreads through the lymphatic system and the blood, and "seeds" the entire immune system, including the large network of lymph nodes, thymus gland, skin, mucous membranes, and the central nervous system (brain and spine). We can usually detect HIV-viral RNA or DNA within two weeks of infection, and HIV antibodies usually appear within a month or two of initial infection. Virus levels during Acute HIV infection are very high, commonly exceeding one million copies of HIV RNA for every milliliter of blood [*see Figure 4*].

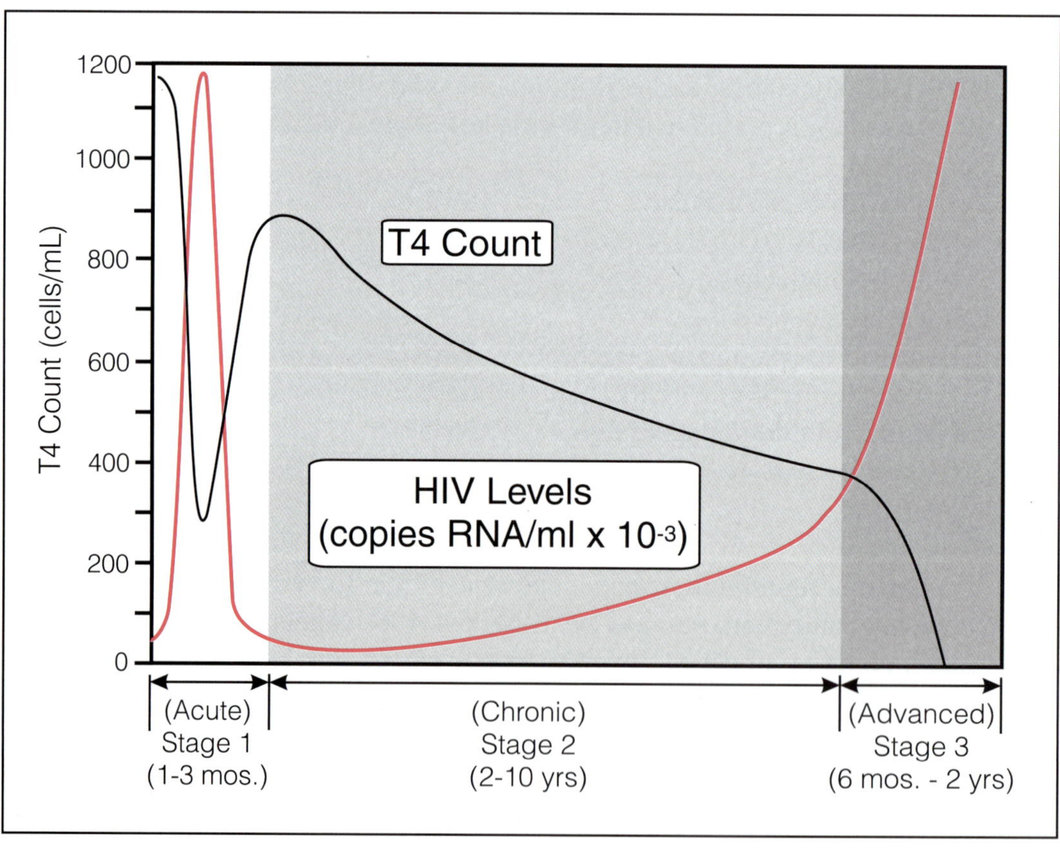

Figure 4 **HIV rises rapidly [red line] and then declines during Acute HIV, then slowly returns causing continuous damage during Chronic HIV, and replicates out of control during Advanced HIV.**

Although people typically don't know they have HIV during Stage 1, because of the exceedingly high levels of HIV present in blood, tissue, and semen during this period, they are highly contagious.

STAGE 2: CHRONIC HIV INFECTION

Stage 1, Acute HIV Infection, usually resolves on its own, and the infected person returns to a feeling of normal health, with the exception of a few enlarged lymph nodes. Stage 2, Chronic HIV Infection, spans the next two to 10 years, during which there may be no notable clinical events and the infected person wouldn't know he had any medical problems, unless specific laboratory tests were performed that revealed HIV infection. In this stage I have heard reports of tiredness or fatigue. Weight loss may occur, but is rare and usually mild.

During Stage 2, the only infection that occurs at a higher frequency in people with HIV than in people without HIV is Zoster (Shingles), which is a limited recurrence of Chickenpox. This occurs in 5% to 10% of people with HIV infection per year, and shows up as a large painful cluster of blisters that wraps from the spine or back of the head around the body to the mid-line of the other side. Because this infection follows the pathways of nerves, it only occurs on one side of the head or body at a time. Pain may be mild, but in most cases Zoster is very painful and can cause permanent nerve damage and scarring.

HIV does **not** become dormant during the chronic stage. Slowly and progressively reproducing itself 10 billion times a day everyday, it becomes heavier in the lymph nodes and other structures of the immune system. It may have begun infecting 10% to 20% of lymph nodes and dendritic cells, but as the years progress, HIV steadily invades 50%, and then 80% to 90% of all one's lymph node tissue and dendritic cells. The level of HIV infection becomes deeper and more entrenched. The ability of the body to make millions of new T4 cells to replace those destroyed becomes more difficult. And while a drop in the T4 cell count of 75 to 100 points per year may not seem like a precipitous depletion, ultimately, the battle shifts in the favor of HIV, and the T4 count slides steadily lower.

Many doctors and researchers used to believe that HIV was quiescent during Stage 2, and recommended holding off therapy until Stage 3. Now it is clear that HIV is chronically and steadily active during Stage 2. In fact this is the stage in which most of the damage is being done to the infected person. Today we have radically changed our approach. Now we try aggressively to stop HIV from damaging the immune system during all stages.

The Higher the HIV Viral Level, the More Rapidly a Person Becomes Ill

The ability to measure the level of HIV infection in a person at any given time is now measurable by blood tests using one of two techniques, either HIV Quantitative RNA PCR, or HIV Quantitative b-DNA. We had assumed for years that the higher the activity of HIV, the more rapidly a person's immune system would be damaged, and the more rapidly that person would progress to severe illness. We could not have been more correct. Furthermore, we now know that if a person has a high HIV viral level that is reduced or, better yet, driven to zero (undetectable) by effective triple therapy, that person's health and survival will improve greatly.

The most classic study followed 181 people with HIV over a period of five to 10 years, measuring viral levels approximately every six months. Data on HIV viral level and median time of progression to AIDS are shown below:

If one's HIV Viral Level is:	One develops AIDS in:
less than 4500	8.0 years
4500 to 13000	6.5 years
13000 to 36000	4.5 years
more than 36,000	2.5 years

Data on the progression from Stage 3 to death demonstrates similar results. People with higher HIV viral levels die at a much higher rate than those with lower HIV viral levels. The good news is that additional studies have now shown that if one lowers HIV viral levels, health stabilizes and death rates drop dramatically. Even more interesting studies are underway to evaluate the effect of a zero or undetectable HIV viral level on quality of life and longevity. Preliminary information indicates the possibility of a return to normal health.

STAGE 3: ADVANCED HIV INFECTION OR AIDS

Without proper therapy, virtually all people infected with HIV progress to Stage 3, also known as Advanced HIV Infection or AIDS. During this stage, the T4 count rapidly drops to very low levels or zero, and without any counter force, the virus soars, often rising above one million copies of HIV per milliliter (one half teaspoon) of blood. Viral levels are 100 to 1000 times higher in Stage 3 than during

Stage 2 infection, and what little remains of the immune system is rapidly destroyed. In *Figure 4*, one can see the rapid rise of HIV and the corresponding rapid decline in T4 cells that occurs during Advanced HIV Infection. Like a snowball rolling downhill, HIV in Stage 3 replicates out of control, and what little remains of the immune system is overwhelmed. Now the infected person is vulnerable to many potentially lethal infections and cancers. If he or she fails to obtain proper medical treatment to prevent these infections and to suppress HIV replication, one or more serious infections are likely to occur within six months, and the individual will probably die within six months to one year.

The most common infections during Stage 3 are:

- **Herpes** (Simplex) infection of the mouth, esophagus, and genitals,
- **Zoster** (Shingles),
- **PCP** (Pneumocystis carinii pneumonia),
- **Candida** infection of the mouth and esophagus,
- **Cryptococcus** infection of the brain lining, lungs, and blood,
- **MAI** (Mycobacterium avian intracellulare) of the blood, lung and liver,
- **Toxoplasmosis** of the brain, lung and muscle,
- **CMV** (Cytomegalovirus) infection of the eye, lung, brain, spine, esophagus, and colon.

The most common cancers are **lymphoma**, and **Kaposi's Sarcoma**, although Kaposi's Sarcoma is now considered a viral sarcoma (slow growing tissue), not a true cancer.

Untreated, HIV infection is one of the most debilitating and lethal infections ever discovered. Some facts that we have covered are summarized below.

- **HIV rapidly infects and kills T4 cells,** and chronically infects macrophages and dendritic cells,

- **HIV is chronically active**, with no dormant state,

- untreated, **HIV causes progressive, unrelenting damage** to the immune system,

- **immune systems** that are infected by HIV **appear permanently damaged** (although some early research indicates that with proper treatment, some immune system repair may be possible),

- **HIV changes (mutates) rapidly**, evading the immune system,

- because of the high mutation rate of HIV, **single therapy is useless**, and **two drug combinations are of limited use,** and

- **untreated, more than 95% of persons with HIV infection die** within two to fifteen years of becoming infected.

HIV is an impressive and complex virus that untreated causes debilitation and death unparalleled by previously studied human infections. Our knowledge of the virus and the disease it causes is extensive. Given this knowledge, it makes only good common sense to attack this infection as early as possible with the most comprehensive therapy available. Virtually all people with HIV infection die of the disease if effective treatment is not provided.

4
MEDICINES TO TREAT HIV INFECTION

4 MEDICINES TO TREAT HIV INFECTION

In this chapter, we'll look at the sites of HIV replication and the classes of medicines that have been developed thus far to halt the virus. The goal of each of these medicines is to block a specific step of replication of HIV. Success is measured by a decreased HIV viral load. People with HIV infection whose HIV viral levels are consistently zero or undetectable by our most sensitive methods of testing are considered in **Remission**, and will experience a return to normal or near normal health, with a corresponding increase in T4 count. This is because proper therapy shuts off the HIV infection, allowing the immune system to return to a normal functioning state. As the immune system becomes stronger, patients feel better and experience improved energy, appetite, and sense of well being. The operable word above is "proper" therapy—the appropriate application of the medicines that can make a difference in HIV replication—by which we mean triple therapy.

TRIPLE THERAPY RAPIDLY SHUTS OFF HIV

Triple therapy is applied over a period of four to six weeks in the form of **Drug A**, then **Drug A + Drug B**, and finally **Drug A + Drug B + Drug C**. The therapy is introduced sequentially and in rapid succession to allow patient and doctor to evaluate each drug for one to two weeks for effectiveness and lack of side effects. Effectiveness is measured by comparing the HIV viral level before and after the addition of the medicine. This is called **"Comparison PCR."** An effective drug is one which causes the HIV Quantitative RNA PCR to drop more than 50% (preferably 80-90%) in a two week period. Drugs that are effective and cause no significant side effects for the patient stay in the therapy. Those that are ineffective or produce significant side effects are thrown out and alternative medicines are substituted. With effective triple therapy, HIV viral levels frequently reach zero or undectable by week four taking **Drug A + Drug B**, and almost always reach zero by week six taking **Drug A + Drug B + Drug C**.

THE IMMUNE SYSTEM SLOWLY IMPROVES

However, the immune system is a large organ. It is not surprising that the T4 count does not rise rapidly in response to rapidly lowered HIV viral levels. The count didn't drop rapidly in response to the onslaught of HIV either. The T4 response to any change in HIV viral level begins within one to two months and stabilizes by about month three or four. Typically in triple therapy, T4 cells increase during the first few months and then again between years one and two. In months one through three HIV is cleared out of the T4 Cell Compartment. Between years one and two, HIV is cleared from the Latent Cell Compartment.

It is not surprising to see the immune system improving in two phases corresponding to the clearance of HIV from the two compartments. Further, research using biopsies of lymph node tissue, gastrointestinal tissue, and spinal fluid is now demonstrating that with triple therapy and sustained zero HIV levels (Remission), 95% or more of HIV can be cleared from the body in one to two years of continuous therapy. Additional research using lymph node biopsies demonstrates signs of immune system repair for the first time.

HIV REPLICATES IN THREE MAJOR PHASES

As shown in *Figure 1,* in **Early Phase** cell binding, penetration, uncoating, and reverse transcription occur. In **Mid Phase** integration, transcription, and translation take place. **Late Phase** includes assembly, budding, and maturation. As discussed in Chapter 2, HIV binds to the T4 cell in **Step 1: cell binding**. HIV enters the T4 cell in **Step 2: penetration**, and removes its fatty outer coat in **Step 3: uncoating**. In **Step 4: reverse transcription**, HIV transforms its genetic code from RNA to DNA, than inserts this new HIV DNA into the human genes in **Step 5: integration**. In **Step 6: transcription**, the HIV DNA activates to produce hundreds of copies of HIV RNA, which is converted to protein sequences in **Step 7: translation**. **Steps 8 through 10** include the **assembly** of the newly forming HIV, the **budding** process through the T4 outer membrane, and their **maturation** to infectious, mature HIV by the activity of HIV protease.

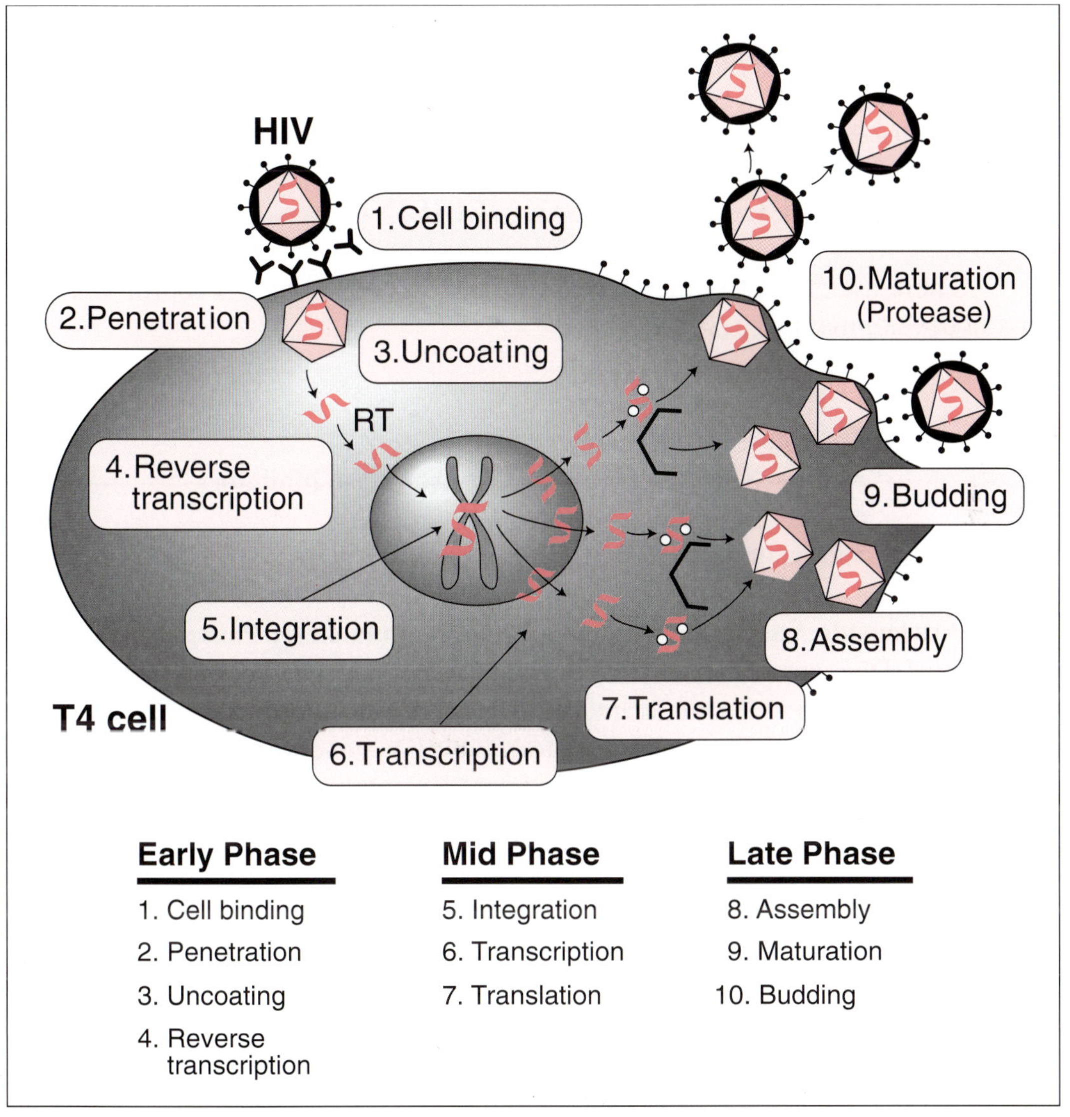

Figure 1 **HIV replicates in three phases: Early Phase, Mid Phase, and Late Phase and 10 major steps.**

FINDING THREE EFFECTIVE MEDICINES

Our goal is to find, for each person, **three medicines** that completely and permanently shut off HIV infection, thus halting the disease process. Medicines need to be chosen based on each case, ideally to address each of the different phases and different steps of HIV replication.

Each medicine must fit two criteria. Each medicine must be effective on its own, as measured by a minimum of 50% decrease (preferably 80%-90% decrease) in HIV viral level over a two week period when the drug is first taken. And each medicine must be free of significant side effects in each case.

THE DIFFERENT CLASSES OF HIV MEDICINES

There are currently three classes of HIV medicine, and a fourth and fifth class in development. These are:

1. Nucleoside Analogs
2. Protease Inhibitors
3. Non-Nucleoside Reverse Transcriptase Inhibitors
4. Integrase Inhibitors (in development)
5. Fusion Inhibitors (in development)

Nucleoside Analogs block HIV replication in its Early Phase replication by binding to HIV reverse transcriptase and through chain termination in Early and Mid Phase replication. From Chapter 2, reverse transcriptase is an HIV chemical that performs the "retro" step by transforming HIV genetic code RNA to DNA. Chain termination is the blockage of the formation of new HIV RNA "chains" by the medicines known as Nucleoside Analogs.

Protease Inhibitors are medicines that block HIV replication in Late Phase by binding to HIV protease, which stops maturation of newly formed HIV virus.

Non-Nucleoside Reverse Transcriptase Inhibitors (NNRTIs) are another class of medicines that block HIV in Early Phase by binding to reverse transcriptase.

A new class of HIV medicines in development is called **Integrase Inhibitors.** These medicines block HIV replication in Mid Phase by binding HIV integrase. HIV integrase is a chemical produced by HIV that allows HIV DNA to integrate or become part of human genes. By blocking this step, medicines in this family halt the HIV replication process by preventing the HIV genetic code from entering the T4 cell genetic code, thus stopping the replication process from moving forward.

Fusion Inhibitors, also in development, block HIV in Early Phase by blocking HIV fusion to the T4 cell membrane.

Each class of medicines is effective in blocking HIV replication at a specific phase and step of its cycle [*see Figure 2*].

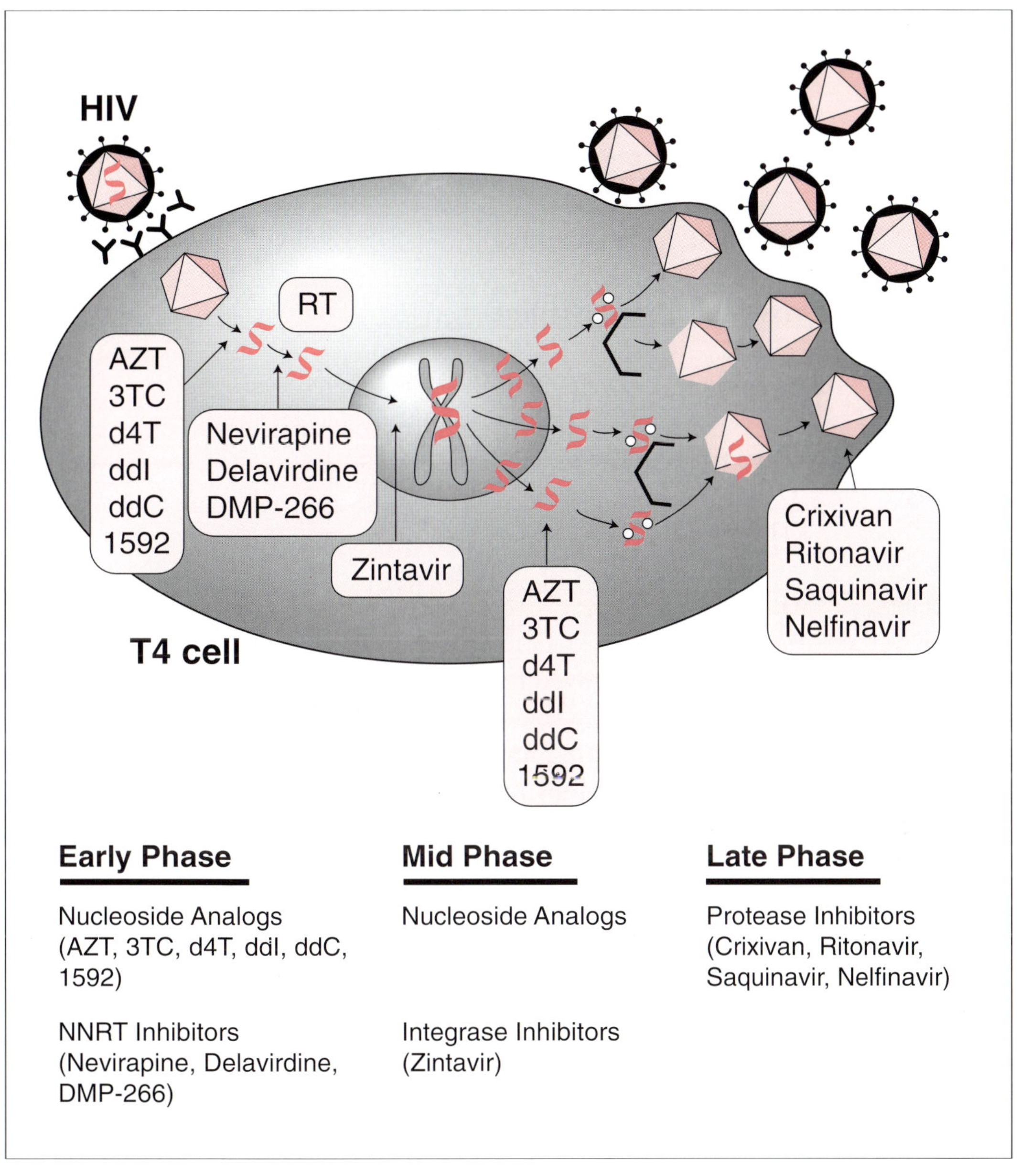

Figure 2 **The HIV replication cycle and the location and phase where each class of medicines and each particular medicine blocks HIV from replicating.**

There are numerous medicines within each of these five classes of HIV medications [*see Table 1*].

Table 1 **The classes of HIV medicines and the individual medicines approved or in advanced stages of research testing.**

Nucleoside Analog	Protease Inhibitor	Non-Nucleoside RT Inhibitor	Integrase Inhibitor	Fusion Inhibitor
AZT	**Saquinavir**	**Nevirapine**	*Zintevir	*Pentafuside
ddI	**Crixivan**	**Delavirdine**		
ddC	**Ritonavir**	*DMP-266		
3TC	**Nelfinavir**	*Loviride		
d4T	*141W94	*MKC-442		
*1592U89	*ABT-378			

* In development and not yet approved for use by the FDA

Many more are under testing, and some have entered early human trials. *Table 2* lists additional HIV medicines in early planning or development, which if successful in early research, may advance to further research trials and move on to FDA approval in 1998 or 1999.

Let's continue by describing some important aspects of these classes of HIV medicines, followed by a short description of each individual medicine.

NUCLEOSIDE ANALOGS

Many of the HIV medicines currently available are in the family of medicines named Nucleoside Analogs. These medicines are derived from the four building blocks (nucleosides) of our genetic code, DNA (Deoxyribose Nucleic Acid). The four building blocks for DNA are:

A - Adenosine, **C - Cytidine,**
T - Thymidine, **G - Guanosine.**

The difference between DNA and RNA (Ribose Nucleic Acid) is that RNA is composed of U-Uridine and not T-Thymidine; but its other components, A, C, and G, are the same as those of DNA.

Table 2 **Other possible HIV medicines "in the pipeline" some of which may move to further research and approval while others may fail early research.**

Name	Target/Type of Medicine
Azodicarbonamide	Nucleocapside Zinc Finger
CP-51	Fusion Inhibitor
CN1-Ho294	Nuclear Translocation
CL-1012	NC p7
Fp-21399	Cell Entry
GEM-91	Gag mRNA
ISIS-5320	gp120 V3 Loop
NSC-687025	Post Transcription Target
Adefovir (BisPOM-PMEA)	Nucleotide Analog
BM 21.1290	
CS92	
DADP	
FTC	

THE COMPUTER CODE OF LIFE: A, C, T, G

DNA and its sister molecule, RNA, are the "computer code of life," forming the genetic material of most living organisms. Whereas computers use a binary code of 1 or 0 to code data, biologic computer data is coded in a quaternary code of A or T (or U) or C or G to code genetic data. DNA and RNA are made of long repeating sequences of these building blocks [*see Figure 3*].

Human cells (and HIV) use these four building blocks: A, T (or U), C, G, to make new sequences of genetic material for new human cells (and for new HIV virus). However, human cells have very specific enzymes and techniques that allow them to distinguish A, T, C, and G from other similar substances, while HIV is generally **unable** to distinguish between the building blocks of DNA and other similar compounds. Because HIV lacks the sophistication of human cells in this aspect of its replication cycle, researchers realized this as an area of vulnerability for HIV. Taking each of the four building blocks of DNA, they began modifying them one at a time.

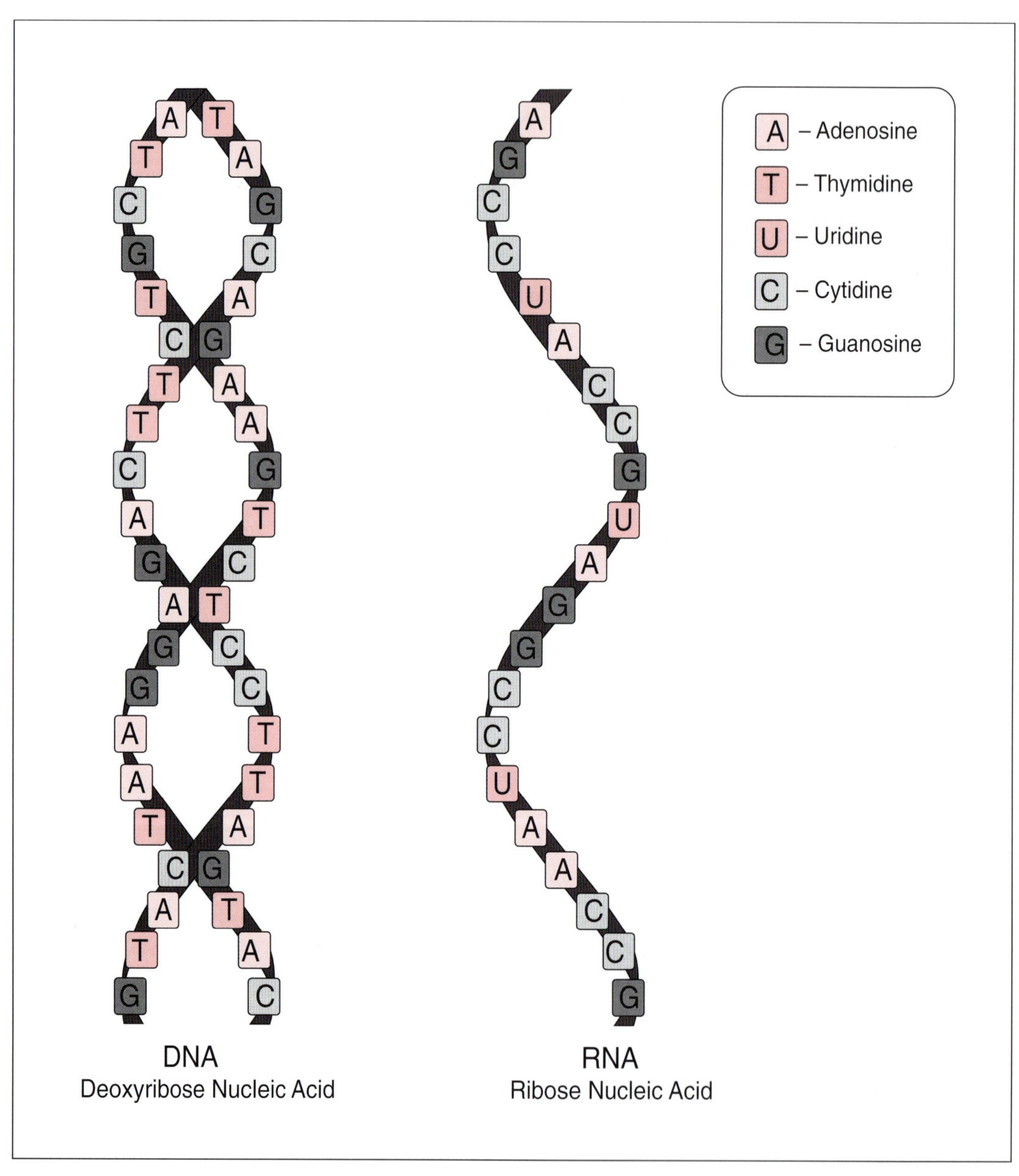

Figure 3 **DNA appears as a two-stranded coil on the left, with its sister molecule, RNA (Ribose Nucleic Acid), as a single strand on the right. DNA is made of the building blocks A, T, C, G and RNA is made of A, U, C, G.**

THE DISCOVERY OF AZT

The goal was to develop a slightly modified nucleoside that the human cell would ignore (and therefore not be harmed by), but that HIV would attempt to use in its replication cycle. Thousands of compounds were screened. In 1986 one such modified nucleoside was discovered that did not seem to significantly harm human cells, but did shut off HIV replication. This compound used a nucleoside T (thymidine) modified to Azidothymidine, or **AZT** for short.

FURTHER DEVELOPMENT OF ddI, ddC, 3TC, d4T, & 1592

As AZT went to human tests, the hunt continued for other safe modified nucleosides or **nucleoside analogs**. Soon thereafter, a modified nucleoside A (Adenosine), called ddA was found, which proved too fragile to be effective, but it led researchers to a related compound, **ddI**, or dideoxyinosine, which is converted in human cells to ddA, and with further intracellular modifications inhibits HIV replication. After AZT and ddI came two modified nucleosides of C (Cytidine), **ddC** and **3TC**, and another modified nucleoside of T (Thymidine), **d4T**. In development is a promising modification of G (Guanosine), which may reach pharmacies in 1998. It is compound **1592U89**, recently named **Abacavir**.

Nucleoside Analogs are a very powerful class of antiviral medicines. In binding to reverse transcriptase in Early Phase HIV replication, they prevent the reverse transcription of HIV RNA to HIV DNA. If some HIV DNA begins to be made, Nucleoside Analogs cause chain termination of the DNA sequencing by preventing binding of the next nucleoside in the chain. Without this step, HIV cannot proceed to infect the nucleus of human cells, and replication stops. Unfortunately, this binding step is reversible. Nucleoside Analogs can float up to reverse transcriptase and bind to it. However, they can also unbind and float away, allowing reverse transcriptase to function again.

Nucleoside Analogs also inhibit HIV replication in Mid Phase transcription. If HIV is transcribed from RNA to DNA and inserts itself into the human cell nucleus, it may attempt to make hundreds of HIV RNA copies. In this step, if the RNA picks up a modified C (Cytidine), say ddC, the ddC locks onto the previous building block, but does not permit the addition of the next building block. In essence, the Nucleoside Analogs lack the "hooks" to form a chain, which causes "chain termination" of HIV RNA and an end to the replication process [*see Figure 4*].

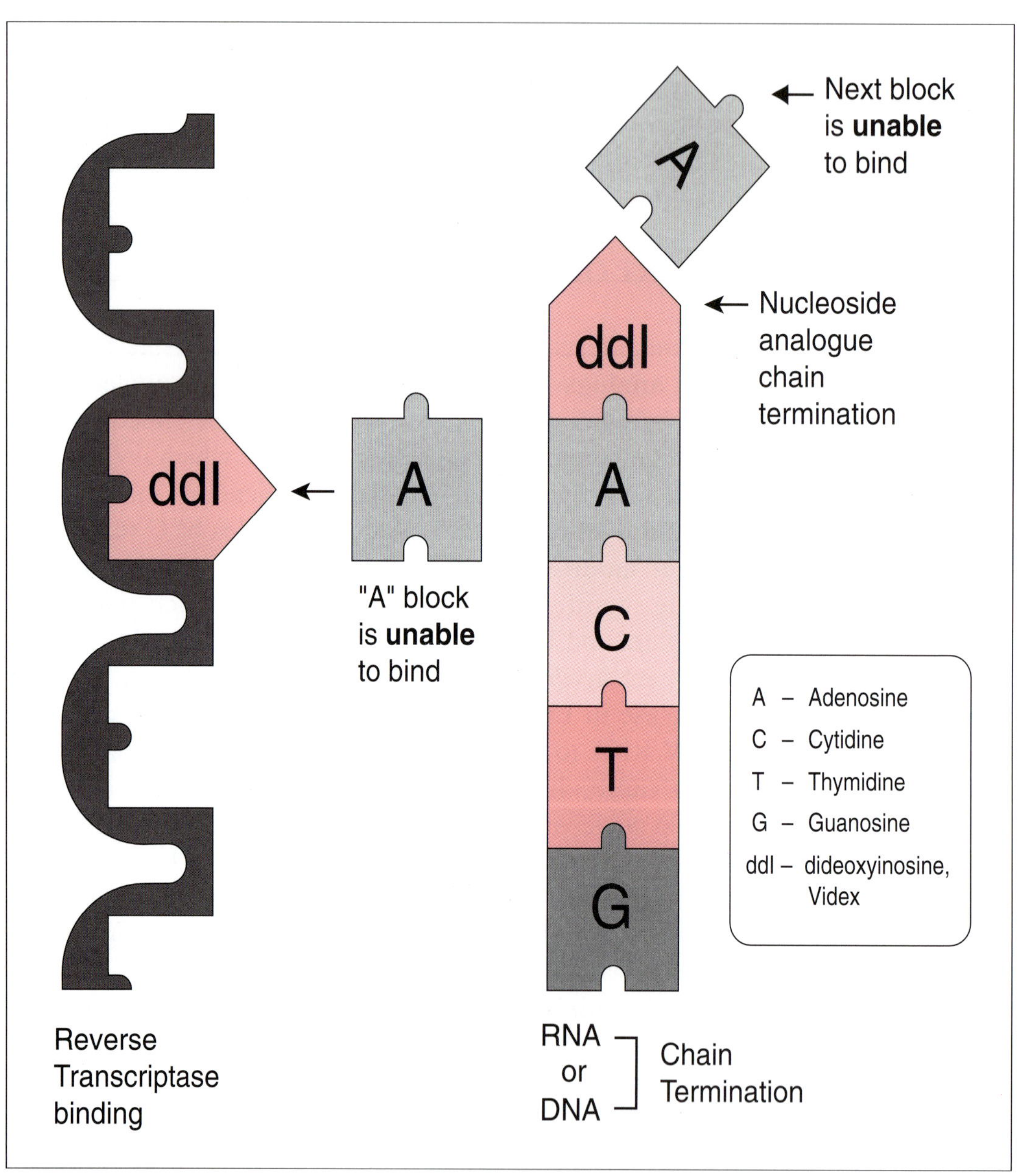

Figure 4 **The HIV medicines called Nucleoside Analogs (AZT, d4T, ddI, ddC, 3TC, 1592) inhibit HIV replication by binding reverse transcriptase and by causing "chain termination" of new elongating strands of HIV RNA or HIV DNA.**

MEDICINES IN THE NUCLEOSIDE ANALOG FAMILY

AZT (RETROVIR)

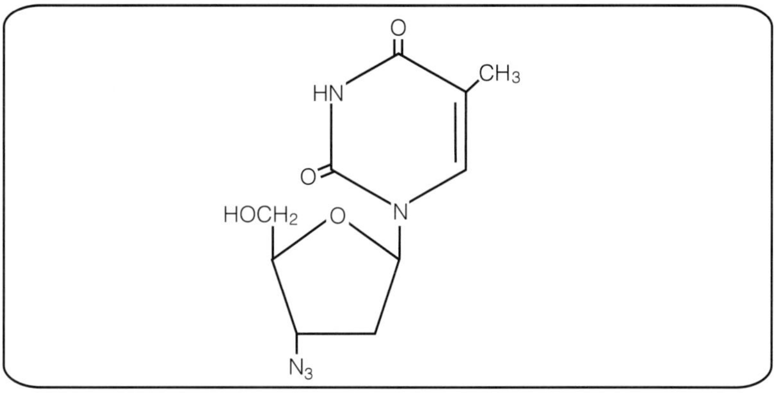

Name: AZT, Azidothymidine, Retrovir, Zidovudine
Structure: 3'azido3'deoxythymidine, thymidine analog
Class: Nucleoside Analog
Mechanism of action: RT inhibitor and chain termination
Dosing: (100mg or 300mg tablets) 200mg to 300mg twice per day with food
Side effects: (30%) headache, nausea, fatigue, anemia, neutropenia, myositis
Manufacturer: GlaxoWellcome

Figure 5 **The molecular structure and information for AZT.**

AZT, also known as **Azidothymidine, Zidovudine,** and **Retrovir**, is an HIV medicine derived from the nucleoside T (Thymidine) [*see Figure 5*]. Initially discovered at the National Institutes of Health as a possible anti-cancer drug, AZT was further developed by BurroughsWellcome Pharmaceuticals (now Glaxo-Wellcome) as the first medicine shown to inhibit HIV replication in the lab. Being the first of the anti-HIV medications ever developed, it still forms the core of many combination and triple therapies, and many new medications are compared to AZT for their relative effectiveness. As an HIV medicine, its potency is moderate, and like any single therapy developed to date, the virus forms resistant strains unaffected by AZT after six to 12 months, if used as single therapy. Single therapy should never be used for more than two to four weeks. In combination or triple therapy, AZT's effectiveness is measured in years, with some treatments lasting more than four years to date, and still working. Approximately 70% of people tolerate AZT without significant problems. In the remaining 30% there may be side effects including lowered white count, lowered red count (anemia), fatigue, headaches, nausea, vomiting, muscle aches, and malaise.

The medicines derived from the nucleoside T (thymidine), which currently include AZT and d4T, act differently from those that are derived from A (Adenosine), C (Cytidine), or G (Guanosine) nucleosides. The Thymidine derivatives are able to inhibit HIV when the T cell is in a resting state. The other Nucleoside Analogs require that the T cell be in a stimulated or active state to inhibit HIV. Thus, the Thymidine derivatives are considered a different subclass than the other Nucleoside Analogs and complement the others when they are selected as part of a combination or triple therapy.

d4T (ZERIT)

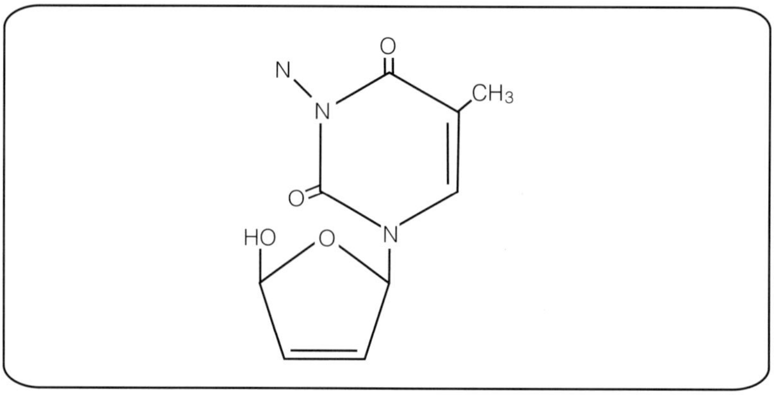

Name: d4T, dihydrodeoxythymidine, Zerit, Stavudine
Structure: 2',3'didehydro3'deoxythymidine
Class: Nucleoside Analog
Mechanism of action: RT inhibitor and chain terminator
Dose: (20mg, 30mg, 40mg capsules) 30mg to 40mg twice per day with food
Side effects: (10%) neuropathy, pancreatitis, fatigue, insomnia, hepatitis
Manufacturer: Bristol-Myers Squibb

Figure 6 **The molecular structure and information for d4T.**

d4T, also known as **Zerit** or **Stavudine**, is a second medicine derived from the nucleoside T (Thymidine) [*see Figure 6*]. As such, it inhibits HIV during rest and non-resting phases of cell replication. Its potency is strong and in recent studies appears more effective than AZT. Like all HIV medications developed to date, it also should only be used in combination or triple therapy to avoid resistance and therapy failure, as single therapy fails in three to 12 months. Limitations on drug dosing come mainly from the high incidence of side effects at doses higher than 40mg twice per day. Approximately 90% of people take this medication with no side effects at all. In the other 10% the most common dose-dependent side effect is nerve damage (neuropathy), occurring mainly as a "stocking glove" distribution numbness, tingling, or pain in the feet and hands. Other rare side effects include liver inflammation (hepatitis), pancreas inflammation (pancreatitis), fatigue, difficulty sleeping, and diarrhea. This medicine can be safely used as first line therapy, for people with side effects to AZT, or for those with resistance to AZT.

ddI (VIDEX)

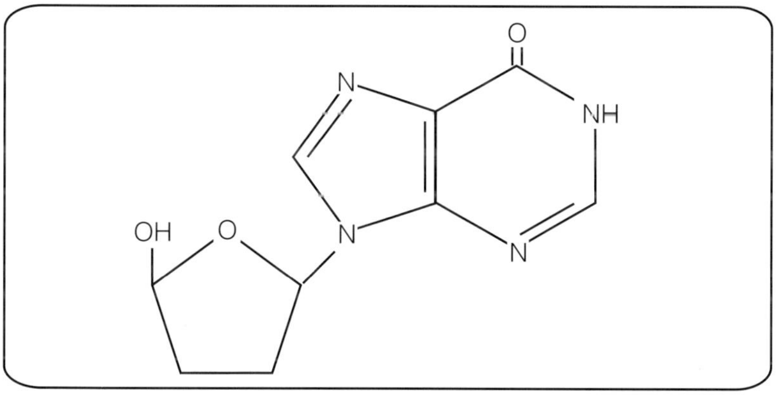

Name: ddI, dideoxyinosine, Videx, Didanosine
Structure: 2',3'dideoxyinosine
Class: Nucleoside Analog
Mechanism of action: RT inhibitor and chain terminator
Dose: (50mg, 100mg, 150mg tablets) 100mg to 200mg twice per day on empty stomach, not to be taken within one hour of other HIV medicines
Side effects: (10%) diarrhea, neuropathy, pancreatitis
Manufacturer: Bristol-Myers Squibb

Figure 7 **The molecular structure and information for ddI.**

ddI, also known as **Videx** or **Didanosine**, is derived from the building block Inosine, of the nucleoside A (Adenosine) [*see Figure 7*]. ddI is the only HIV medicine derived from Adenosine/Inosine developed to date. It was approved in 1991, and is one of the most effective HIV medicines we have. Its usual dose is 200mg twice per day. Resistance in single therapy does not typically develop for more than two years, making this the longest lasting single therapy for HIV so far although it should not be used alone for any case of HIV infection with currently available advanced therapy. In addition it has the longest half life of any HIV medication, consisting of eight to 24 hours. Viral loads typically are reduced 70% to 90% within two weeks of initiating ddI therapy.

Approximately 70% of patients can take ddI without any significant side effects. Loose bowel movements and diarrhea are not uncommon due to the "Mylanta-like" alkaline buffer in ddI. Immodium AD (Loperamide) or Lomotil can be given with ddI to counter this annoying yet relatively harmless side effect.

Neuropathy occurs in less than 10% of cases in the same gradual "stocking glove" distribution of numbness or pain, as it can with d4T or ddC. If ddI is stopped immediately, the symptoms usually resolve within one to two weeks or sooner without permanent problems. However, if dosed too high, or if a person with an early neuropathy continues to take ddI, pain and numbness can advance up the arms or legs and become permanent. Thus, if any signs of neuropathy occur, the patient should stop the medicine immediately and consult with his or her doctor. Like all therapy for HIV infection, close communication between physician and patient are crucial.

Other rare side effects are pancreatitis, tongue soreness, and fatigue. An acidic environment inactivates the drug by converting it to xanthine. Thus ddI is the only currently approved HIV medicine that should be taken on an empty stomach, and no food eaten for 45 minutes to one hour after taking the medicine, which can be somewhat inconvenient. Generally, ddI is very powerful. It can be prescribed safely and with excellent results, if one does not exceed a dose of 400mg per day and if the medicine is stopped if any problems begin. As with all medicines used to treat HIV infection, ddI should only be used in combination (double or triple) to reduce the risk of HIV viral mutations and the development of HIV resistance to ddI.

ddC (HIVID)

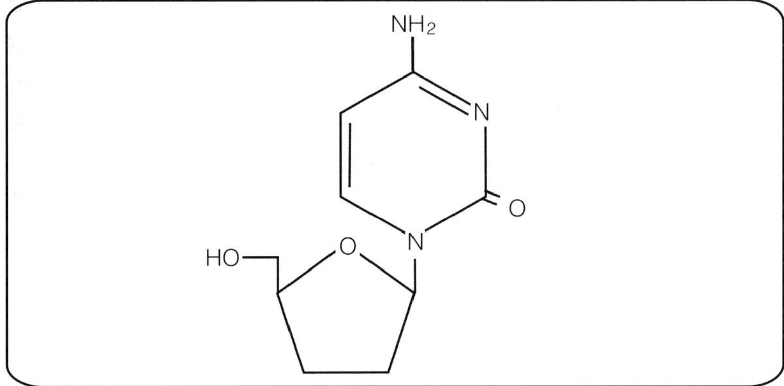

Name: ddC, dideoxycytidine, Hivid, Zalcitabine
Structure: 2',3'dideoxycytidine
Class: Nucleoside Analog
Mechanism of action: RT inhibitor and chain terminator
Dose: (0.375mg, 0.75mg tablets) 0.75mg twice or three times per day with food
Side effects: (10%) oral ulcers, neuropathy, hepatitis, fatigue, pancreatitis
Manufacturer: HoffmanLaRoche

Figure 8 **The molecular structure and information for ddC.**

ddC, also known as **Hivid** or **Zalcitabine**, is the third anti-HIV medicine developed, derived from the nucleoside C (Cytidine). It is the **weakest** Nucleoside Analog approved to date because it must be taken in very low doses (1.5mg to 2.25mg per day). These dosage limitations were established during clinical trials. Although a potent drug against HIV in the test tube, in clinical trials higher doses of ddC failed in humans because of their side effects: nerve damage (neuropathy), pancreas inflammation (pancreatitis), liver inflammation (hepatitis), and oral ulcers. Due to the extreme limitations on dosing I do not recommend using this drug in therapy unless there is no alternative. It is doubtful that the tolerable dose is sufficient to saturate the lymphoid tissue of the immune system. Furthermore, in clinical trials resistance to ddC can be rapid, and ddC always finishes last in effectiveness compared to other HIV medicines.

3TC (EPIVIR)

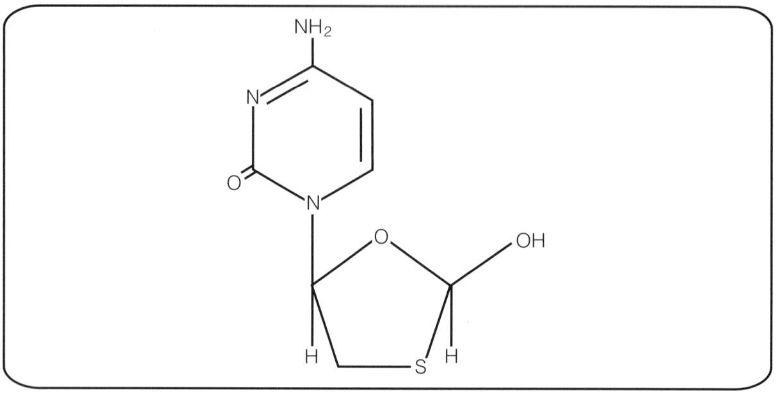

Name: 3TC, dideoxythiacytidine, Epivir, Lamivudine
Structure: (-)2',3'dideoxy,3'thiacytidine
Class: Nucleoside Analog
Mechanism of action: RT inhibitor and chain terminator
Dose: (150mg tablets) 150mg twice per day with food
Side effects: (2%) hepatitis, neuropathy, hair loss, fatigue
Manufacturer: GlaxoWellcome

Figure 9 **The molecular structure and information for 3TC.**

3TC, also known as **Epivir** or **Lamivudine**, is derived from Cytidine, as is ddC. This is the safest HIV medicine yet developed. Some very rare side effects are hair loss, hepatitis, neuropathy, fatigue, mouth sores, and diarrhea. However, most people who take 3TC have no side effects at all [*see Figure 9*].

3TC almost didn't make the cut for FDA approval. In early research HIV resistance occurred rapidly, by week four to eight in most cases. However, when combined with other nucleosides, especially the Thymidine group (AZT or d4T), 3TC forms a powerful block of HIV replication and sustains it. The reason for this prolonged effect, especially given the early research data, is not clear.

In any case, the combinations of **AZT + 3TC** or **d4T + 3TC** are some of the most effective, safe, and easily administered therapies for HIV infection. One can expect more than 95% of people to tolerate one or the other without problems. They form the "backbone" of our best triple therapies. When the third part of the triple therapy, a Protease Inhibitor, is added, most cases go into Remission.

3TC is administered twice per day with or without food. Dosing in adults is always 150mg twice per day. Higher doses produce no additional benefit. 3TC has also been found to be effective against Hepatitis B virus.

***1592 (ABACAVIR)**

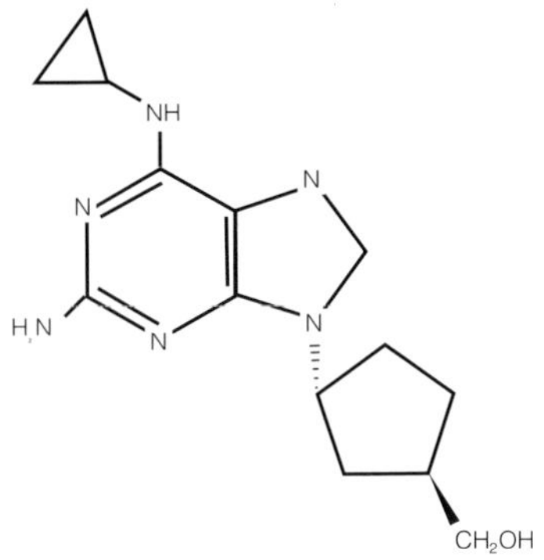

NH
N
N
H_2N
N
N
CH_2OH

Name: 1592, 1592U89, Abacavir
Structure: Carbocyclic Guanosine Nucleoside
Class: Nucleoside Analog
Mechanism of action: RT inhibitor and chain terminator
Dose: 300mg twice per day (currently in research testing)
Side effects: (10% to 20%) nausea, headache, diarrhea
Manufacturer: GlaxoWellcome
*not yet approved by the FDA

Figure 10 **The molecular structure and information for 1592 (Abacavir).**

1592, also known as **1592U89** or **Abacavir**, is the first successful HIV medicine that is derived from the nucleoside G (Guanosine) [*see Figure 10*]. In early research, 1592 appears to safely and effectively suppress HIV replication. It does this so well, that it is at least twice as strong as any other Nucleoside Analog developed to date, and compares in strength to the newer Protease Inhibitors. Other derivatives of Guanosine are Acyclovir and Ganciclovir which are only effective in suppressing viruses in the Herpes virus family.

1592 is the most exciting and promising nucleoside that we've seen during the past 10 years. Preliminary research shows that 1592 suppresses HIV 100 fold, and has a resistance pattern different from all other medicines studied. It potentially combines well with other Nucleoside Analogs, NNRTIs, and Protease Inhibitors. It is a very important new HIV medicine because of its effectiveness, relative safety, and most importantly its unique structure compared to other nucleosides. This means that people who have become resistant to such common HIV medicines as AZT, d4T, ddC, ddI, and 3TC, should respond favorably to 1592 with a Protease Inhibitor such as Nelfinavir, or 1592 with a NNRTI such as DMP-266, or 1592 plus Nelfinavir plus DMP-266, and they could begin their therapy again. GlaxoWellcome, the pharmaceutical company that owns 1592, has begun phase 3 research trials with 1592. If research continues at its present pace, it is unlikely that 1592 will be FDA approved prior to 1998. However, people failing current therapies have a pressing need for 1592. I must urge GlaxoWellcome to form a special Expanded Access Program to allow such people to receive 1592 prior to its formal approval, as has been done in previous HIV medicines while they were under development.

PROTEASE INHIBITORS

The second major class of HIV medicines is the **Protease Inhibitors**. Proteases are unique chemicals contained in many viruses that process proteins of newly formed viruses, thereby converting these virus from immature, non-infectious forms to mature, infectious virus. Proteases do not exist in human cells, thus medicines, such as Protease Inhibitors, that bind and block protease enzymes should not cause any direct harm to people who take them. The HIV protease is a chemical, specific to HIV, that cuts and processes proteins of immature HIV virus and converts these newly formed HIV to mature, infectious HIV. Without Protease, HIV might produce new HIV virus, but they would be nonfunctional, unable to infect new T4 cells. As their name implies, Protease Inhibitors bind to and inhibit HIV-specific protease from performing its function.

When the HIV protease molecule was recognized in the late 1980s, a number of large pharmaceutical companies went to work to design and build medicines to inhibit its function. Four medicines in the Protease Inhibitor family, the first class of HIV medicines successfully designed and chemically constructed by research pharmaceutical companies, are now FDA approved for use in fighting HIV infection. Two additional protease inhibitors will likely be approved by 1998. With the success of this new class of medications, we have entered the new and rapidly evolving era of "designer drugs" and drug development. It's a whole new world, unlike the random evaluation and testing of existing substances as occurred with the Nucleoside Analogs.

SAQUINAVIR (INVIRASE)

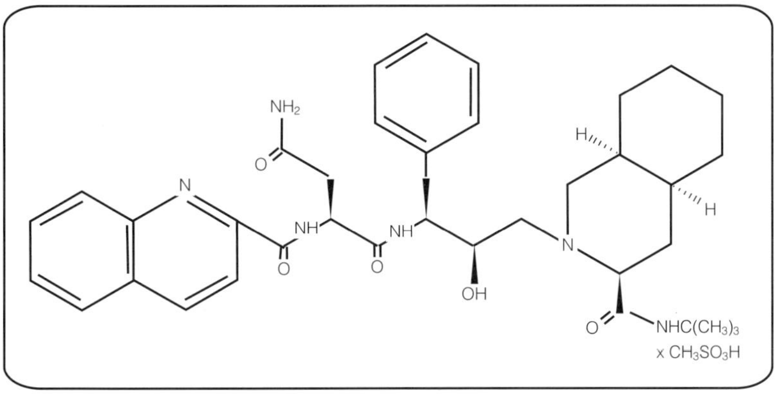

Name: Saquinavir, Invirase, Saquinavir mesylate
Structure: N-butyl-decahydro-2-isoquindine-3s-carboxamide-methanesulfonate
Class: Protease Inhibitor
Mechanism of action: inhibits HIV protease thereby inhibiting HIV maturation
Dose: (200mg capsules) 1200mg to 1800mg three times per day with food
Side effects: (20%) nausea, bloating, diarrhea, headache
Manufacturer: HoffmanLaRoche

Figure 11 **The molecular structure and information for Saquinavir.**

Saquinavir, or **Invirase**, was the first Protease Inhibitor produced and approved by the FDA in late 1995. This drug is well tolerated without side effects in approximately 80% of patients [*see Figure 11*]. Occasionally nausea, headaches, fatigue, and diarrhea are reported. There is a significant problem with Saquinavir, however. **The medicine is only 4% absorbed.** This means that with each pill taken, 96% goes through the intestines directly into the toilet. This makes Saquinavir a very weak medication for HIV, with frequent treatment failure. Newer studies have indicated that **the FDA approved dose of 600mg (three pills) taken three times per day is too low** a dose to effectively suppress HIV replication. Research studies suggest that the minimum effective dose of Saquinavir is 1200mg (six pills) taken three times per day and that perhaps 1800mg (nine pills) taken three times per day might be even better. But it is unreasonable to ask anyone to take this huge number of pills per day for a marginal benefit at best. Thus, unless no other options exist, most experienced physicians treating HIV, myself included, have put Saquinavir aside until the absorption problem is fixed by the company that makes it. HoffmanLaRoche is currently working on a new formulation that is 20% absorbed. I look forward to the new formulation; unfortunately, HoffmanLaRoche hasn't said when it might be available.

Resistance can occur with Saquinavir as with any other HIV medication used to date. Saquinavir resistance usually occurs within six months, especially if it is used improperly as single therapy. Remember, single therapy should never be used to treat HIV infection (see Chapter 5). As with most resistance, once a person's HIV strain is resistant to Saquinavir, that medication will probably never work for that person for the rest of his or her life. A disturbing finding has been that some people who become resistant to Saquinavir have reduced response or no response to other Protease Inhibitors. Given these complex issues, until the new formulation of Saquinavir is available, I recommend that other more effective Protease Inhibitors be tried first. In its current form Saquinavir should be used only as a back up treatment, and then only at a dose of six to nine pills three time per day.

INDINAVIR (CRIXIVAN)

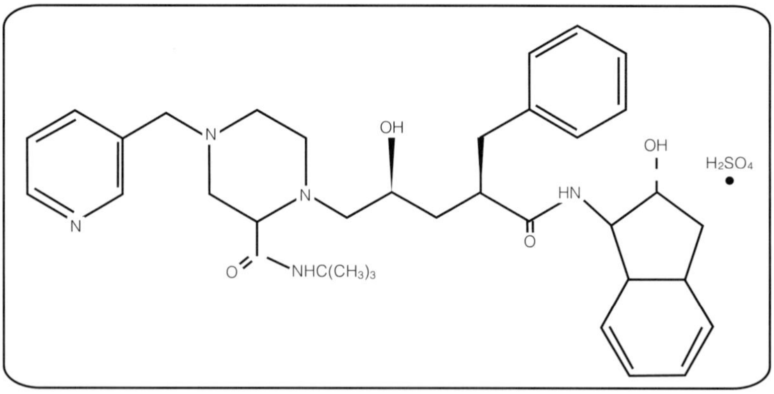

Name: Crixivan, Indinivir
Structure: 2,3,5-tridoexy-N-5-2-D-erythro-pentonamide sulfate
Class: Protease Inhibitor
Mechanism of action: inhibits HIV protease thereby inhibiting HIV maturation
Dose: (200mg, 400mg) 800mg three times per day on empty or light stomach
Side effects: kidney stones, nausea, fatigue, insomnia, renal failure, hepatitis
Manufacturer: Merck

Figure 12 **The molecular structure and information for Crixivan.**

Crixivan, or **Indinavir**, is one of the safest and most effective Protease Inhibitors [*see Figure 12*]. It was approved in early 1996 after leading physicians and patient advocate groups reviewed early research data and insisted on rapid approval. The FDA responded with the fastest approval of any medicine in U.S. history, 40 days after the application for Crixivan was submitted by Merck Pharmaceuticals.

Crixivan is made in 200mg and 400mg capsules. The recommended dose is two capsules, or 800mg, taken three times per day. Since concurrent protein or fat may reduce absorption by 50%, it is recommended that Crixivan be taken on a light or empty stomach. However, carbohydrates, including breads, cereals, low fat milk, juices, and probably fruits and vegetables may be taken concurrently with Crixivan without reduced effectiveness.

Crixivan's effectiveness in early studies is impressive, with more than 50% of people attaining zero or undetectable HIV viral levels on single therapy and more than 80% attaining undetectable HIV viral levels in triple therapy. As with all HIV medications, Crixivan should never be taken as single therapy, and it is most effective as part of triple therapy regimens. In single therapy research studies, resistance occurred within six months, was complete, and permanent. In triple therapy, effectiveness has been sustained for almost two years now with no signs of failure in most cases.

More than 90% of patients in my experience and in published studies easily tolerate Crixivan without any problems. The most common comment I hear from my patients is how dramatically their health has improved and how much energy they have on a triple therapy that includes Crixivan. Up to 15% of patients may experience transient, mild side effects, including dry eyes, dry mouth, occasional bitter taste, fatigue, headache, or nausea. Approximately 4% of people taking Crixivan develop kidney stones, primarily presenting as left or right flank pain, with occasional dysuria (pain while urinating). These stones are a result of Crixivan's poor solubility. Adequate hydration (eight to 10 glasses of liquid per day) prevents most occurrences. I instruct my patients to drink enough fluid each day so their urine is clear or at least light yellow. If they see that their urine is medium yellow or darker, they need to drink more fluid.

Other rare side effects include an elevated bilirubin (a liver test), hepatitis, or kidney failure. A chemistry test should be done every two to three months and if any side effects occur, one should consider changing to an alternative Protease Inhibitor, such as Nelfinavir.

RITONAVIR (NORVIR)

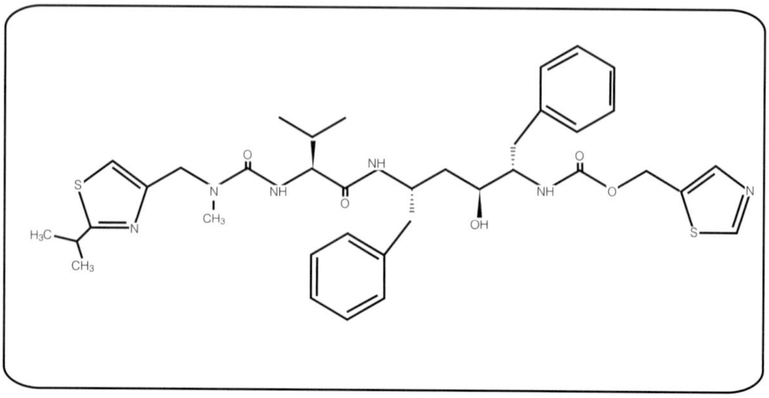

Name: Ritonavir, Norvir
Structure: hydroxy-methyl-dioxo-tetraazatridecan-oic acid-thiazolylmethyl ester
Class: Protease Inhibitor
Mechanism of action: inhibits HIV protease thereby inhibiting HIV maturation
Dose: (100mg capsules) six twice per day with food (keep medicine refrigerated)
Side effects: fatigue, headache, nausea, numbness, hepatitis, liver failure
Manufacturer: Abbott

Figure 13 **The molecular structure and information for Ritonavir.**

Ritonavir, or **Norvir**, is a very powerful Protease Inhibitor developed by Abbott Laboratories and approved by the FDA in early 1996 [*see Figure 13*]. Like Saquinavir and Crixivan, it binds the active site of HIV protease, inhibiting the effect of HIV protease, and preventing the maturation of HIV virions.

Ritonavir is made in 100mg capsules, and the recommended dose in adults is six capsules twice per day with a meal. Ritonavir must be kept refrigerated to maintain its effectiveness. HIV viral levels drop precipitously when Ritonavir is taken, similar to the response seen in people on Crixivan. Resistance develops within six months in the same fashion as for all Protease Inhibitors when they are used alone, by HIV mutation of the protease-active site. Resistance is permanent if it occurs. Single therapy should never be used, and most experienced physicians use Ritonavir as a third and powerful member of an effective triple therapy for HIV infection. Like Crixivan, Ritonavir is most effectively combined with a Thymidine

Nucleoside Analog (AZT or d4T), and a Non-Thymidine Nucleoside Analog (3TC, ddI, or ddC).

The major factors that have kept Ritonavir from wide spread popularity have been frequent and potentially serious side effects, its potential for cross reaction with many other medications, and its high cost—not that most HIV medicines aren't costly. AZT and most Nucleoside Analogs cost approximately $200 per month per drug. Crixivan costs approximately $390 per month. But Ritonavir costs an average of $600 to $700 per month.

Many people who take Ritonavir experience nausea, headache, vomiting, diarrhea, and an unusual numbness, particularly around their mouth and other parts of their body. Some people are so ill while taking this medication that they are unable to function. The manufacturer, Abbott, recognized these problems and has now produced a dosing regiment that starts Ritonavir at a lower dose and gradually increases to full dose within two to four weeks. Sometimes this strategy is successful.

Ritonavir interacts strongly with a processing system of the liver, called the p-450 system. In doing so, any other medicine that is processed through the p-450 system should not be taken with Ritonavir or, if absolutely necessary, a dose modification of the second medication and Ritonavir may be necessary to avoid serious side effects. Additionally, Ritonavir may cause hepatitis or in some rare cases, liver damage, liver failure, and even death.

With its high incidence of potentially severe side effects, its difficulty in combining with other medications, and its higher cost, many experienced physicians have placed Ritonavir second or third as compared to other Protease Inhibitors when prescribing treatments for their patients.

Some interesting new developments with another Protease Inhibitor of Abbott, ABT-378, may predict the future of Ritonavir. Still in research development, ABT-378 appears to be ten times more powerful and much safer than Ritonavir. Abbott is currently testing full dose ABT-378 combined with 50mg of Ritonavir. By forming this combination, Ritonavir greatly increases the blood level of ABT-378, and allows ABT-378 to be taken conveniently twice per day. In addition, this small amount of Ritonavir appears to avoid the significant side effects of a full dose of Ritonavir and boosts the blood levels of ABT-378 so well that the combination ABT-378 + low dose Ritonavir effectively treats HIV that is resistant to Ritonavir, Crixivan, and Saquinavir. Thus, it is likely that Ritonavir may soon become a secondary drug to enhance the effectiveness of ABT-378, rather than continue as a mainstream HIV medicine.

NELFINAVIR (VIRACEPT)

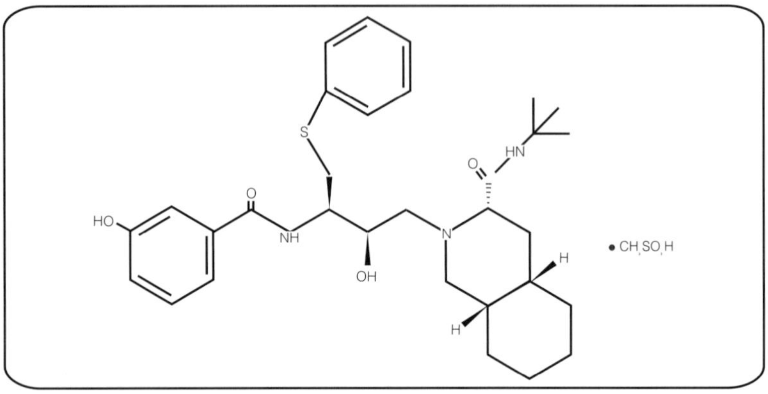

Name: Nelfinavir, Viracept
Structure: N-decahydro-2-3-isoquinolinecarboxamide mono-methanesulfonate
Class: Protease Inhibitor
Mechanism of action: inhibits HIV protease thereby inhibiting HIV maturation
Dose: (250mg tablets) 750mg three times per day with food
Side effects: (20%) diarrhea, nausea
Manufacturer: Agouron

Figure 14 **The molecular structure and information for Nelfinavir.**

Nelfinavir, or **Viracept**, is the newest and the fourth Protease Inhibitor to be approved by the FDA. Its safety profile is excellent and its effectiveness approaches that of Crixivan, making it one of the best HIV medicines developed to date. It is produced in 250mg capsules; the standard adult dose is 750mg three times per day [*see Figure 14*]. A pediatric formula designed for treatment of HIV-infected babies and young children is also available. For more information on pediatric treatment, contact the parent company, Agouron, or a pediatrician experienced in the treatment of HIV-infected children.

Like all HIV medicines developed to date, single therapy Nelfinavir fails rapidly due to resistance by month three to six, and appears irreversible. Nelfinavir-resistant HIV appears to work differently than HIV that is resistant to other Protease Inhibitors: People with Nelfinavir-resistant HIV may benefit by changing to another Protease Inhibitor such as Crixivan, Saquinavir, or Ritonavir. Those resistant to other Protease Inhibitors may benefit by changing to Nelfinavir.

In Phase 2 research trials, AZT + 3TC + Nelfinavir put 80% of people into Remission, as measured by repeated HIV viral levels of zero or undetectable. In this study, T4 levels increased by more than 150 points.

Possible side effects include nausea, diarrhea, and theoretically, liver dysfunction. Nelfinavir is processed by the liver, and should not be given concurrently with drugs that are heavily processed by the liver such as Rifampin, Seldane, or Ketoconazole, without dose adjustments by a physician or pharmacist.

NNRTIs

The **NNRTIs** (Non-Nucleoside Reverse Transcriptase Inhibitors) are medicines that inhibit or bind to reverse transcriptase (RT), thereby deactivating RT and halting HIV replication in Early Phase. Currently two such medicines **Nevirapine and Delavirdine**, have been approved by the FDA.

This class of medicines is an entirely new class specifically designed for treatment of HIV infection. While currently approved NNRTIs are effective in suppressing HIV replication in the lab, they have several major weaknesses:

- their binding of reverse transcriptase (RT) is reversible,
- unlike Nucleoside Analogs which act at two different sites (reverse transcriptase binding and chain termination), the NNRTIs only act at one specific site,
- HIV can invalidate the currently approved NNRTIs through a single mutation,
- As a result, in single therapy, current NNRTIs may fail within two to eight weeks, a shorter time than other medicines developed thus far.

Nevirapine and Delavirdine are the only medicines that have consistently failed in combination therapy and have now been shown to be ineffective in at least one triple therapy. In fact, results from a recent trial show that **Nevirapine + AZT + ddI is no better than AZT + ddI.** In my opinion, although theoretically interesting, this class of HIV medicines does not yet have the sustained benefit or effectiveness to be an active part of a strong, long term triple therapy. In particular, the rapid resistance, and the failure in combination therapy are ominous signs of medicines that will likely have extremely limited use, and may silently fail, thus leading to failure of other parts of an otherwise effective triple therapy. This could in turn lead to multi-drug failure and a multi-resistant HIV strain in some cases.

A new NNRTI under development, DMP-266, appears to overcome these problems. It is highly effective, safe, has a long duration of effectiveness, and requires multiple HIV mutations (rather than a single mutation for Nevirapine and Delavirdine) to form resistance. In my opinion, until DMP-266 is available, Nevirapine and Delavirdine offer little and other more beneficial medicines are currently available and should be considered first before embarking on the use of this class of medicines.

NEVIRAPINE (VIRAMUNE)

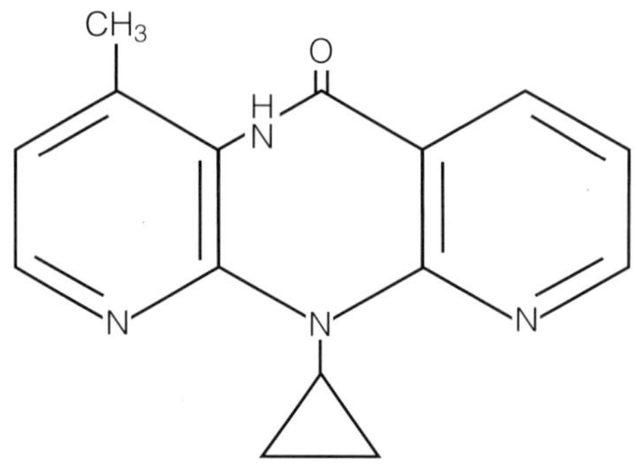

Name: Nevirapine, NVP, Viramune
Structure: 11-cyclopropyl-5,11-dihydro-4-methyl-6H-dipyrido-diazepin-6-one
Class: NNRTI (Non-Nucleoside Reverse Transcriptase Inhibitor)
Mechanism of action: RT inhibitor
Dose: (200mg capsules) one per day for two weeks, then one twice per day
Side effects: (20%) rash, Stevens-Johnson Syndrome, nausea, diarrhea
Manufacturer: Roxane

Figure 15 **The molecular structure and information for Nevirapine.**

Nevirapine, also known as **Viramune** or **NVP**, is the first NNRTI approved for use in HIV infection [*see Figure 15*]. It should never be used in single therapy due to the rapid resistance that occurs within two weeks in almost all cases. Nor should it be used in two drug combination therapy, as studies have recently documented its failure in combination. Even Nevirapine's use in triple therapy regiments is now in question. It should be used with caution if at all.

Like all NNRTIs, Nevirapine acts by reversibly binding reverse transcriptase. However, if HIV mutates, at it routinely does, it may quickly become fully resistant to Nevirapine.

Serious side effects may occur with Nevirapine. The most common is Stevens-Johnson Syndrome or Toxic Epidermal Necrolysis, a potentially lethal syndrome where a poison or a drug rapidly causes the skin and the mucus membranes of the body to die. Patients with severe Stevens-Johnson Syndrome have diffuse redness, followed by blistering and peeling of their skin. This may be so severe that they resemble burn victims. Treatment includes immediately stopping the medicine, administering corticosteroids, fluid hydration, and antibiotics. Severe cases may require Intensive Care Unit or Burn Unit admission. The death rate from severe Stevens-Johnson Syndrome is high.

DELAVIRDINE (RESCRIPTOR)

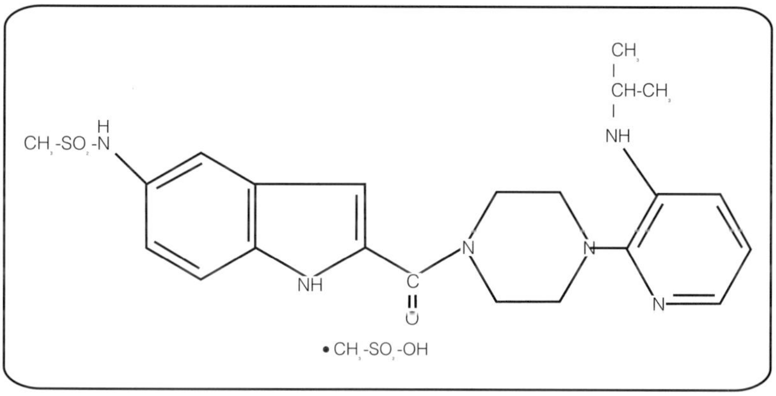

Name: Delavirdine, DLV, Rescriptor
Structure: piperazine, 1-3-2 pyridinyl-4-carbonyl monomethane sulfonate
Class: NNRTI (Non-Nucleoside Reverse Transcriptase Inhibitor)
Mechanism of action: RT inhibitor
Dose: (100mg tablets) four tablets three times per day
Side effects: rash, Stevens-Johnson Syndrome, nausea, diarrhea
Manufacturer: Pharmacia & Upjohn

Figure 16 **The molecular structure and information for Delavirdine.**

Delavirdine, also known as **Rescriptor** or **DLV**, is the second NNRTI approved for the treatment of HIV infection. It is similar in effectiveness and side effects to Nevirapine. One interesting report has indicated that Delavirdine at 400mg three times per day may protect AZT from developing resistance. Further studies are underway.

HIV MEDICINES IN DEVELOPMENT

A number of powerful and interesting medicines are currently in research development for the treatment of HIV infection. Furthermore, the rate of discovery of new compounds is dramatically increasing compared to years past, and with the increasing size of the U.S. and world HIV epidemic, there is a large and growing financial incentive to produce new medicines.

INTEGRASE INHIBITORS

One of the most fascinating new classes of HIV medicines under development is the **Integrase Inhibitors**, the first of which is called **Zintavir**. Integrase is that crucial enzyme which permits HIV DNA to be cut and inserted into the human cell DNA. Without integrase, infection of the human cell does not proceed and HIV replication is impossible. Zintavir has apparently passed Phase 1 trials without any significant side effects and is proceeding to Phase 2 research trials. If successful, this new class of HIV medicines could easily be as successful or more successful than even the Protease Inhibitors. Theoretically, a combination of a Nucleoside Analog, an Integrase Inhibitor, and a Protease Inhibitor could rapidly and completely halt HIV replication. This has the potential to become one of the most powerful and effective therapies developed to date.

FUSION INHIBITORS

A second class of HIV medicines under development is the **Fusion Inhibitors**, the first of which is **Pentafuside**. This new class of medicines is designed to stop HIV from binding to the T4 cell, thus blocking its entry into the cell and halting replication in Early Phase. If successful, this class of medicines could stop infection of any new cells by HIV, making a large and positive impact on the health of a person with HIV infection. Like the Integrase Inhibitors, a combination of a successful Fusion Inhibitor with any of the other classes of HIV medicines could be a very powerful treatment for HIV infection.

NUCLEOSIDE ANALOGS IN DEVELOPMENT

Among the new Nucleoside Analogs under research development, the most promising is compound **1592U89**. Recall that DNA is made of four building blocks, A-Adenosine, T-Thymidine, C-Cytidine, and G-Guanosine. To date, we have developed HIV medicines from the A group (ddI), the T group (AZT, d4T), and the C group (3TC, ddC). 1592 (Abacavir) is a powerful Nucleoside Analog derived from the G group. Preliminary reports indicate that the medicine is well tolerated. HIV viral levels drop by 90% to 99% (10 to 100 fold), making this compound's effect on HIV replication similar to that of the Protease Inhibitors. Some minor side effects of nausea, fatigue, and headache have been reported.

PROTEASE INHIBITORS IN DEVELOPMENT

Protease Inhibitor development is booming. The two most promising in development are **141W94** (also known as **VX-478**) by GlaxoWellcome, and **ABT-378** by Abbott Pharmaceuticals. Both appear highly effective in early studies. Abbott's ABT-378 is ten times more powerful than Ritonavir. Much work remains to be done and approval is not expected until 1998.

NNRTIs IN DEVELOPMENT

Additional NNRTIs in development are **DMP-266, Loviride,** and **MKC-442**. DMP-266 appears to overcome the rapid resistance and failure seen with Nevirapine and Delavirdine. Its development moving ahead quickly and approval may come later in 1997 or 1998.

The list of effective HIV medicines continues to rapidly grow and many more are being developed, expanding the options for people with HIV infection. The next chapter, Chapter 5, will explain the reasoning and methods of combining these medicines into effective triple therapy.

5
TRIPLE THERAPY:
Recipes To Good Health

5 TRIPLE THERAPY:
Recipes To Good Health

CONCEPTS OF TREATMENT: "HIT IT EARLY & HIT IT HARD"

The goal is to provide treatment that allows the immune system to become as strong as possible. The best measure of the strength of one's immune system is the T4 cell count and the individual's ability to avoid or fight infections. When HIV has weakened the immune system, therapy is focused on completely and continuously suppressing HIV replication. We can see how we're doing by measuring HIV viral levels. When HIV infection is completely suppressed, the immune system regains strength and the health of the person with HIV infection dramatically improves.

We've never seen anything quite like HIV. No disease in recent history has caused doctors to formulate so many theories, or people to try such bizarre therapies, such as heating their blood, filling their colons with ozone, or painting their skin with caustic chemicals in an attempt to slow the disease. One must wonder why this disease has caused such chaos in the scientific as well as public community, and why confusion still exists today.

THE FACTS ARE SIMPLE ENOUGH

HIV is an infection that continuously and thoroughly destroys the body's immune system, resulting in sickness and death. **The solution to HIV is also not complicated**: successful treatment requires completely and continuously shutting off HIV replication, for it is only when HIV replicates that it causes sickness and damage. What gets complex is HIV's ability to mutate. HIV is not only a moving target, it is an ever changing moving target.

A few key concepts should be remembered when designing and providing treatment for people with HIV infection:

- **Respect this virus. HIV is tricky and elusive.**
- **Never underestimate this virus.**
- **When HIV is faltering, do not let up. Hit it again.**

.

The only effective way to treat HIV is to treat it as soon as it is discovered in each person, and treat it with the most powerful, effective medicines available. Triple therapy is the **minimum** therapy that fully suppresses HIV.

TRIPLE THERAPY TRULY IS THE GOLD STANDARD

Recent data on the mathematical modeling of HIV infection has shown us that **single and double therapy will fail**, given the replication rate of HIV and its ability to continuously mutate to different forms. There is also some new, very exciting news about triple therapy:

- Triple therapy that includes a powerful Protease Inhibitor is able to quickly put most people with HIV into Remission, as confirmed by a zero or undetectable viral level.
- In Remission, if the HIV viral level stays at zero, at least three separate studies now confirm that 90% to 95% of HIV can be cleared from the body over a period of one to two years.
- Effective triple therapy shows no signs of failure for up to the length of the studies, which are now beyond the three year mark.

The only failures of triple therapy, according to the latest research, have been among those patients who had taken one of the study medicines (AZT) for a prolonged time prior to beginning the triple therapy. It is likely that these cases were unsuccessful due to preexisting resistance. When we say resistance, we mean an HIV infection that has adapted to a medicine so that the medicine no longer works against it. In the cases of Remission on effective triple therapy, only about 5% of the HIV infection remains after one to two years of therapy. This remaining HIV is integrated, dormant HIV DNA hidden within human genes through the integration step of HIV replication. Until a cure is found, people with HIV must continue taking triple therapy to prevent HIV from reseeding the immune system from this small, remaining HIV DNA. Our cure projects will now be focused on ridding the body of this remaining HIV material.

PROBLEMS WITH THE CURRENT HIV TREATMENT GUIDELINES

There is a huge void in leadership in the field of HIV treatment and in the national management of the HIV epidemic. There actually are **no** national HIV treatment guidelines to direct physicians on how to treat HIV disease. The most current recommendations published in the Journal of the American Medical Association (JAMA) in July 1996 are vague and already out of date [*see Figure 1*].

Figure 1 **Summary of the Current Published Recommendations for Primary and Established HIV Infection.**

> **PRIMARY INFECTION:** The panel, although suggesting the enrollment of patients in controlled clinical trials, recommended the treatment of primary infection with the most potent combination available — at least two Nucleoside Analogs plus, if available, a Protease Inhibitor or a Non-Nucleoside Reverse Transcriptase Inhibitor (NNRTI) — for a minimum of six months.
>
> **ESTABLISHED INFECTION:** Initiation of Therapy: Initiation of therapy is recommended for all symptomatic patients and for asymptomatic patients with CD4 cell counts of 500 or less. Initiation of therapy is recommended for asymptomatic patients with more than 500 CD4 cells and HIV RNA plasma levels over 30,000 copies, or a rapidly declining CD4 cell count. The panel recommends initiation of therapy be considered for asymptomatic patients with CD4 cell counts over 500 and HIV RNA plasma levels over 5000 to 10,000 copies.
>
> **Choice of Therapy:** The panel recommends initiation of therapy with a minimum of two Nucleoside Analogs (evidence exists to support the ddI monotherapy option, although it is less strong than for combination therapy). The panel considers it a reasonable option to start with one of the most potent combinations available, e.g., one that includes a Protease Inhibitor, which can be selected primarily for anti-retroviral potency, secondarily for safety, tolerability, and drug resistance pattern.

AN EPIDEMIC IS A NATIONAL CRISIS

We have lost more than 350,000 people nationwide, and more than 10 million worldwide. People are still dying. **Guidelines need to be direct and clear.** They should include the most up-to-date research data and intelligently extrapolate into the future, not hold on to past mistakes.

Such guidelines as currently exist [*see Figure 1*], although much improved from prior guidelines, are long out-of-date. They still list single therapy as an option, when we have more than six years of data showing that **all single therapy produces**

resistance and treatment failure. Furthermore, they encourage patients and physicians to treat HIV with different therapies, recommending no therapy, single therapy (ddI), combination therapy, or triple therapy in different situations. **HIV is an infection that is contained long term only by aggressive triple therapy.** The confusing "soft approach" listed in the guidelines leads to multi-resistant HIV strains and treatment failure. Once a person is resistant to one medicine, that medicine and perhaps other similar medicines likely will never be effective for that person for the rest of his or her life. Furthermore, if we were to follow the JAMA guidelines as currently written, it is likely that over one to two years, many hundreds and even thousands of people with HIV would develop multi-resistant HIV, leading to widespread treatment failures, rapid progression to AIDS, and ultimately widespread death.

The evolution of guidelines for treating HIV has shown a pattern of overcaution and repetitive failure [*see Figure 2*].

Figure 2 **The Evolution of HIV Treatment Guidelines**

Year	Therapies	Guidelines	Status	Number Dead
1981	None	Observe	Failed	200
1984	None	Observe	Failed	5,000
1987	AZT	AZT if T4 less than 200	Failed	40,000
1992	AZT, ddI, ddC	AZT if T4 less than 200, consider AZT if T4 less than 500 and symptoms	Failed	200,000
1996	AZT, ddI, ddC, d4T, 3TC, Crix, Ritonavir, Saquinavir, Nelfinavir, NVP,DLV	Single, double or triple therapy if T4 less than 500, or if symptoms, or if viral level greater than 30,000. Rx if new infection.	Failing	350,000

THE REASONS FOR 10 YEARS OF FAILED GUIDELINES

What is the reason for all these years of overly conservative, vague, and iterative guidelines that have globally failed to help people with HIV infection? Because all of the guidelines for treatment since 1981 were and still are written primarily by Oncologists, physicians whose expertise is in treating cancer, not infections.

How did Oncologists rather than Infectious Disease specialists become the international directors of HIV policy? In the early 1980s the initial presentations of HIV infection were patients who had enlarged lymph glands, called lymphadenopathy. Prior to the discovery of HIV, this symptom was more often a sign of a cancer, such as lymphoma. Thus, primary care doctors, when they encountered these growing numbers of patients with lymphadenopathy, automatically sent them to Oncologists for biopsies of their abnormal lymph glands. In addition, a substantial number of the early cases of HIV and AIDS had an infectious sarcoma, called Kaposi's Sarcoma. Other people came down with a true and typically lethal cancer of the immune system, called lymphoma. And still others had a variety of hematologic complications such as low white counts (neutropenia), low red count (anemia), and low clotting cell levels (thrombocytopenia or ITP), conditions typically managed by the Hematology/ Oncology groups. It didn't take long for the Oncologists to become the experts and managers of large groups of patients with HIV infection, and they continue to be the policy makers of the HIV field today.

DOCTORS OF ONCOLOGY MAY BE FINE PHYSICIANS

However, compared to other fields of medicines, Oncologists specialize in a unique group of patients. It's not surprising that, generally speaking, their treatment philosophy differs from other fields of medicine in that:

- treatment is usually very conservative,
- they do not generally expect cures,
- treatment protocols are by consensus and are adhered to very strictly,
- cancers are "staged" by severity, early being Stage I, more advanced Stage II and Stage III, and most advanced Stage IV,
- most patients are expected to die of their disease despite the best therapy.

The Oncology approach to treatment has been similar to a legal approach. The physician reviews past pertinent cases and treatment protocols, and treats current cases strictly within these guidelines. Compared to other fields of medicine and surgery, you might say Oncologists are somewhat pessimistic about new therapies.

IN COMPARISON IS THE FIELD OF INFECTIOUS DISEASES

Physicians in this field manage infections and tend to have a treatment philosophy dynamically opposite that of the Oncologists. In the field of Infectious Diseases treatment tends to be:

- treat aggressively,
- expect a cure in almost all cases,
- treat based on past protocols, but be innovative and try new concepts, if an infection is not responding,
- each infection is viewed as one entity, treated aggressively whether localized or widespread, and not "staged" as in Oncology,
- expect most patients to live and recover to good health.

The fact that Oncologists became and continue to be the caretakers of all aspects of HIV management and policy has had a profound and, one must conclude, a paralytic effect on the development of treatment guidelines for HIV infection. **It is astounding to realize that it took 10 years of international arguing for the world forum to agree that HIV is an infectious disease** and should be treated as an infectious disease, not as an immune disorder. Furthermore, we have also known for more than six years that HIV mutates faster than almost any other human infection ever discovered. **However, single therapy, which always fails in any mutating infections, was recommended as primary therapy for HIV and AIDS until mid-1996.** Even today, there remain large blocks of physicians and policy makers who are surprised that suppressing HIV infection returns most people to normal health. Indeed, some internationally known leaders in the field still maintain and teach a "wait and see approach" towards therapy.

For infections that do not change or mutate, single medication therapy is usually sufficient. However, **mutagenic infections typically require at minimum two simultaneous medications, and usually three simultaneous medications to effectively suppress the infection and prevent breakthrough with resistant strains.**

THE "CANCER MODEL" DOES NOT FIT HIV

Oncologists formed their field of HIV treatment after the "cancer model" by staging HIV as if it were a cancer, treating it conservatively and by observation, and viewing new advances with great skepticism. But infections are not staged. If they are relatively harmless rhinoviruses, like the common cold, with a low likelihood of serious complications or death, and resolve without therapy, then no therapy or simple supportive therapy is appropriate. However, if an infection is highly damaging or lethal, like Ebola virus, or Lassa fever, or HIV, therapy is urgent and efforts must be made to begin therapy as soon as the infection is detected. **Wait and see is not an option.**

Nor should single therapy be an option. Single therapy has been proved absolutely useless in numerous research protocols. And now we know that combination therapy with two agents is of limited use due to the rapid mutations HIV produces on an ongoing basis. **The only therapy that makes sense is to treat all cases, at all times with a minimum of triple therapy, with the goal of completely and continuously suppressing HIV replication.** Therapy guidelines short of this fail to take into account the basic facts of HIV infection and are doomed to failure. Thus, the new therapy guidelines are "Treat Early, Treat Hard."

HIV infection is a large spectrum disease, and should be treated early, mid and late in the disease, in Stages 1, 2, and 3, with no holds barred. The best therapy is aggressive triple therapy the moment the infection is discovered, and never let up. Any therapy less than this has been proven to fail, and in failing produces resistance, and in so doing permanently eliminates treatment options for the individual. With the current immense volume of research data, everyone with HIV infection should be encouraged to move to triple therapy **immediately**. See my Recommended Revised HIV Treatment Guidelines below in *Figure 3*.

Figure 3 **Recommended Revised and Simple HIV Treatment Guidelines.**

Treat All People with HIV Infection with Aggressive Triple Therapy:

T4 COUNT	HIV VIRAL LEVEL	STAGE OF HIV	THERAPY
all levels	all levels	not applicable (all patients, all stages)	Triple therapy

*The treatment goal is to completely and continuously shut off HIV infection as measured by a zero or undetectable HIV viral level. Some cases may require four drug therapy (the preferred HIV PCR should be accurate to 20 copies/ml).

WHY NOT SINGLE THERAPY?

Single therapy is the administration of a single medicine as treatment for a person with HIV infection. With many infections in medicine, single therapy works very well. For instance, when a person has Strept throat, Penicillin alone is given for one or two weeks with excellent success. How does this work? The Streptococcal bacteria replicate in the throat causing tissue destruction, and covering the throat with more Strept bacteria as the infection advances. In general, Strept bacteria do not mutate or change, or if they do it is very rare. So when Penicillin is given, it kills all the Strept bacteria at one time, as all are identical, and all are susceptible to the action of Penicillin.

In the mid 1980s we thought that single therapy would work against HIV as it does against Strept bacteria. But by the late 1980s it became very apparent that the situation was much more complex. HIV is a retrovirus that mutates, or changes, at an incredible rate. In the process of making more virus, HIV may vary as much as 30% to 60% from the original virus. Many of the new mutant HIV viruses are inactive. However, many others are very functional. The mutations (changes of HIV) occur continuously and randomly. Almost any combination of changes is possible, and given time and no treatment or inadequate treatment, will occur.

Single therapy will always fail to be effective in HIV therapy because HIV will eventually mutate, become resistant to and break through any medicine used as single therapy. Many studies have been completed during the past 10 years documenting the failure of single therapies in HIV infection [*see Figure 4*].

WHY IS DOUBLE OR COMBINATION NOT ENOUGH?

Combination therapy is the administration of two medicines simultaneously in an attempt to halt HIV replication. Although it doesn't last, each single therapy, at its most effective level, is able to lower HIV replication by at most 90%. The combination of two medicines simultaneously should lower HIV replication by more than 95%, but as with single therapy, does not sustain this effectiveness.

Combination therapy has these limitations:

- combination therapy incompletely suppresses HIV infection,
- the benefit of combination therapy only lasts from six months to two years. After that HIV may break through as a multi-resistant strain, unresponsive to either medicine,

- combination therapy is generally able to slow the spread of HIV and halt its progression, but it does not clear the virus from the immune system and usually does not lead to significant immune system improvement,
- eventually HIV breaks through the combination and one progresses to AIDS unless other medicines are available and used.

Figure 4 **Single Therapies and Time to Treatment Failure (Resistance).**

THERAPY	TYPE	TIME TO FAILURE
AZT	Thymidine Nucleoside	6 to 12 months
d4T	Thymidine Nucleoside	6 to 12 months
ddI	Non-Thymidine Nucleoside	12 to 36 months
ddC	Non-Thymidine Nucleoside	6 to 12 months
3TC	Non-Thymidine Nucleoside	4 to 8 weeks
Crixivan	Protease Inhibitor	3 to 6 months
Ritonavir	Protease Inhibitor	3 to 6 months
Saquinavir	Protease Inhibitor	3 to 6 months
Nelfinavir	Protease Inhibitor	3 to 6 months
Nevirapine	NNRTI	2 to 4 weeks
Delavirdine	NNRTI	2 to 8 weeks

Combination or double therapy was our first successful therapy that improved the immune system and health of people with HIV infection [*see Figure 5*]. Although it led to higher quality life and longer survival, the benefits were not permanent—until the discovery of the more powerful Protease Inhibitor class of medicines, which brought us to triple therapy.

Figure 5 **Currently available combination therapies have limited usefulness and lead to multi-resistant HIV infection unless augmented by a Protease Inhibitor*.**

Thymidine Nucleoside		Non-Thymidine Nucleoside
1. **d4T**	+	**3TC**
2. **AZT**	+	**3TC**
3. **d4T**	+	**ddI**
4. **AZT**	+	**ddI**
5. **AZT**	+	**ddC**
6. ——		**ddI + 3TC**

*The combinations are listed in order of the most safe and effective to those that are less effective, from number one to six.

THE MOVE TO TRIPLE THERAPY

Triple therapy is the simultaneous administration of three effective medicines. It is the mainstay in the field of Infectious Disease to treat infections that mutate rapidly. Our best example of another mutating infection, besides HIV, that is successfully treated with triple therapy is the bacterial infection known as Tuberculosis.

Tuberculosis is one of the most common bacterial infections in the world, affecting more than one billion people worldwide at any given time. Until the 1950s it remained untreatable. At first physicians tried single therapy with no success.

Then a couple of insightful doctors tried double therapy with good improvement. Ultimately a three drug regimen, or triple therapy, emerged as the most successful therapy for Tuberculosis. This therapy has stood the test of time for more than 40 years.

There are several reasons why triple therapy works for mutating infections such as Tuberculosis and HIV:

- most infections cannot replicate while being hit by three separate attacks at one time,
- if an infection, like HIV, cannot replicate, it cannot mutate,
- if HIV cannot mutate, it cannot become resistant,
- if it cannot become resistant, it remains shut off,
- as long as HIV is shut off, the therapy remains effective without modification,
- no damage occurs to the immune system,
- and if there is no damage occurring, one's health remains normal.

Mathematical modeling tells us that triple therapy should last almost indefinitely. Given its replication and mutation rate the chances of HIV producing three simultaneous mutations is almost impossible.

A SOFT APPROACH LEADS TO SERIAL RESISTANCE

However, a key point needs emphasizing here. Many patients have been on single therapy for a long time, then been given a second medicine, and then after another while a third medicine. Such a soft, slow approach frequently results in HIV developing a resistance to the first medicine, then the second, and finally to the third. I call this "Serial Resistance." People who have had this type of serial therapy are likely to fail triple therapy within three to six months of adding the third drug. The patient ends up with a multi-resistant HIV infection, and very few options.

For successful triple therapy, each medicine used must be individually effective, so that all three suppress HIV when the therapy is begun. If one is uncertain about any part of the triple therapy, the case should be analyzed by use of an HIV Sensitivity Assay (if available and accurate) or, until then, Comparison PCR (see Chapter 6). When in doubt, change to a completely new triple therapy with medicines that the person has never taken before, to maximize success for the long term.

EFFECTIVE TRIPLE THERAPY CLEARS 95% OF HIV INFECTION

It appears that triple therapy that includes a Protease Inhibitor as one of the three medicines not only halts the spread of HIV in the immune system tissue, but it can permit the body to clear 90% to 95% of its HIV infection over a one to two year period.

Not only does effective triple therapy halt the further spread of HIV in a person, but it actually reverses the disease, and basically allows the body to "clean house" until all that remains of the infection is a small amount of HIV DNA, which we do not yet know how to remove. Not only that—there are currently more than 18 potentially effective triple therapies available, enough to find one to fit every person with HIV infection [*see Figure 6*].

WHY NOT FOUR DRUG OR FIVE DRUG THERAPY?

If three drug therapies are better than two drug therapies, why not use four or five drug therapies? As further research proceeds, we may develop and come to recommend even stronger treatments such as four drug therapies that attack early, mid, and late phase replication, such as:

d4T + 3TC + *Crixivan + Nelfinavir, or

AZT + *1592 + *DMP-266 + Crixivan, or

*1592 + *DMP-266 + *Zintavir + Crixivan

*1592, DMP-266, and Zintavir are currently in research testing and are not FDA approved. The Crixivan + Nelfinavir is conceptual and is scheduled to undergo research testing in the near future.

But it is very probable that three drug therapies will be the mainstay of HIV therapy for most cases until the cure is found, and four drug therapies will only be used by people whose HIV infection is so extensive that three drug therapies only provide partial suppression. Historically, three powerful drugs overwhelm almost any mutating infection. However, if a person begins with a partially resistant strain, or if one or more of the medicines in his or her therapy is not very effective, a four drug therapy might well be the answer.

Figure 6 **Available triple therapies in order of effectiveness & safety.**

Thymidine Nucleoside		Non-Thymidine Nucleoside		Protease Inhibitor	NNRTI
1. **d4T**	+	**3TC**	+	**Crixivan**	
2. **AZT**	+	**3TC**	+	**Crixivan**	
3. **d4T**	+	**3TC**	+	**Nelfinavir**	
4. **AZT**	+	**3TC**	+	**Nelfinavir**	
5. **d4T**	+	**ddI**	+	**Crixivan**	
6. **d4T**	+	**ddI**	+	**Nelfinavir**	
7. **AZT**	+	**ddI**	+	**Crixivan**	
8. **AZT**	+	**ddI**	+	**Nelfinavir**	
9. **AZT**	+	**ddC**	+	**Crixivan**	
10. **AZT**	+	**ddC**	+	**Nelfinavir**	
11. ——		**ddI + 3TC**	+	**Crixivan**	
12. ——		**ddI + 3TC**	+	**Nelfinavir**	
13. **d4T**	+	**3TC**	+	**Ritonavir**	
14. **AZT**	+	**3TC**	+	**Ritonavir**	
15. **d4T**	+	**ddI**	+	**Ritonavir**	
16. **AZT**	+	**ddI**	+	**Ritonavir**	
17. **AZT**	+	**ddC**	+	**Ritonavir**	
18.		**ddI**	**Crixivan + Nelfinavir** (research)		

A four drug therapy has been necessary in **less than 5%** of my cases such as those with:

- a starting T4 count of less than 50,
- multi-resistant HIV strains that are not fully responding to triple therapy,
- high starting HIV viral levels (greater than 500,000 copies/ml).
- active viral levels despite the best triple therapy.

Triple therapy will work in most cases. However, when full suppression is not attained by a three drug therapy, and changing to a more powerful triple therapy is not an option, one must be creative, and do whatever is sensible to maintain the patient's immune system and health. Four drug therapies are new [*see Figure 7*] and there is much yet to learn. The goal is always Remission as measured by a zero (undetectable) HIV viral level.

Figure 7 **Possible four drug therapies for difficult to treat cases of HIV.**

Triple Therapy	**Add Fourth Drug as:**
d4T+3TC+Crixivan	**add ddI**
AZT+3TC+Crixivan	**add ddI**
d4T+ddI+Crixivan	**add 3TC**
AZT+ddI+Crixivan	**add 3TC**
d4T+3TC+Nelfinavir	**add ddI**
AZT+3TC+Nelfinavir	**add ddI**
d4T+ddI+Nelfinavir	**add 3TC**
AZT+ddI+Nelfinavir	**add 3TC**
any with Ritonavir	***add Saquinavir**
any with Crixivan or Nelfinavir	***add Nelfinavir or Crixivan respectively**

*The Ritonavir + Saquinavir and Crixivan + Nelfinavir combinations are undergoing research testing. More data will be available as clinical trials proceed.

THE PROTEASE-PROTEASE COMBINATIONS

As the number of available Protease Inhibitors increases, new combinations of medicines are possible. Two Protease Inhibitors, Ritonavir and Saquinavir, have been used in combination with impressive results. However, Ritonavir causes frequent serious side effects, and Saquinavir is poorly absorbed and needs reformulation. In addition, Ritonavir and Saquinavir have similar resistance patterns. By this I mean that if a person becomes resistant to one of these medicines, they may become resistant to the other without ever having taken it. This is called "cross resistance."

On the other hand, Crixivan and Nelfinavir are individually the most powerful and the safest Protease Inhibitors developed to date. They also have different resistance patterns, making HIV cross resistance against them less likely. Although preliminary data indicates that dose adjustments may be necessary in combination, use in my practice has suggested that both drugs should be maintained as three times per day dosing, and Nelfinavir should be kept at full dose (750mg three times per day) for this combination to be effective. It is not yet clear whether Crixivan should be maintained at full dose (800mg three times per day) or reduced to 600mg three times per day. Futher testing is scheduled by Agouron to answer these questions.

Another possible Protease-Protease combination is Nelfinavir + Saquinavir. Both are taken with meals three times per day making dosing somewhat easier that some other therapies. Neither of these medicines significantly affects liver processing. Thus, I would estimate that for the combination to be effective, both Nelfinavir and Saquinavir would be taken at full doses--Nelfinavir-750mg three times per day and Saquinavir-1200mg three times per day.

The Protease-Protease combinations are new and little testing has been completed. If used in therapy, these combinations would be most effective when combined with one or two additional medicines such as with AZT+3TC, d4T+3TC, AZT+1592, AZT+ Delavirdine, ddI+d4T, or other effective combination therapies. Until further data is available they should not be used as first line therapy, and if used in any case, the physician should contact the pharmaceutical companies for additional instructions on dosing, effectiveness, and any possible side effects.

INITIATING TRIPLE THERAPY

Beginning therapy is straight forward. All new cases should be treated the same way. Remember, the goals are **safe therapy, effective therapy, and an HIV viral level of zero** or undetectable. Use the most accurate and sensitive measurement for HIV viral level available. I suggest using the "Ultrasensitive" HIV Quantitative RNA PCR with a sensitivity to 20 copies/ml. Currently there are 11 HIV medicines approved for use [*see Figure 8*].

Figure 8 **A Review of the Current HIV Medicines and Doses**

Medicine	Type	Dose	Frequency
AZT	**Nucleoside**	**200-300mg**	**twice/day**
d4T	**Nucleoside**	**40mg**	**twice/day**
ddI	**Nucleoside**	**200mg**	**twice/day***
3TC	**Nucleoside**	**150mg**	**twice/day**
ddC	**Nucleoside**	**0.75mg**	**twice or three times/day**
Crixivan	**Protease Inhib.**	**800mg**	**three times/day****
Ritonavir	**Protease Inhib.**	**600mg**	**twice/day**
Saquinavir	**Protease Inhib.**	**1200mg**	**three times/day**
Nelfinavir	**Protease Inhib.**	**750mg**	**three times/day**
Nevirapine	**NNRTI**	**200mg**	**twice/day**
Delavirdine	**NNRTI**	**400mg**	**three times/day**

*For **ddI**, avoid food or Crixivan within 1 hour before or after taking it.
For **Crixivan, avoid meats or fats within 1-2 hours of taking it, it may be taken with carbohydrates (breads, cereals, etc.), drink plenty of fluid, enough to maintain urine color clear or light yellow, spread the three doses widely across the day, early AM, mid afternoon (3 to 5pm), and at bedtime.

RECIPES FOR TRIPLE THERAPY

Following are two examples of triple therapy designed especially for two different circumstances. First for a person who has never taken any HIV medicines [*see Figure 9*] and second for a person beginning triple therapy who has had prior treatment [*see Figure 11*].

Figure 9 **A recipe for triple therapy for a previously untreated case of HIV infection.**

You will need:

d4T or AZT

3TC

Nelfinavir or Crixivan

a good lab with an HIV PCR sensitive to 20 copies/ml

On initial visit, complete a full physical exam including current symptoms, past medical history, allergies, current medicines, vaccination history, places lived, job type, exposure to Tuberculosis, vital signs, and weight. Send the following labs: T cell panel, HIV viral level (HIV Quantitative RNA PCR), Chem 20, CBC/diff, RPR, Hep A, B, C serologies, and Toxoplasma IgG. If there has been any risk of TB, place a TB skin test and read it in two days.

On return visit in two weeks, review the labs with the patient and graph the T4 cell count and HIV viral level on the patient's T4/HIV graph [*see Figure 10*]. Confirm that HIV infection exists by a positive HIV viral level (if unsure, withhold further therapy and send an HIV antibody test). Then initiate medications as follows:

d4T 40mg one twice/day for one week, **if no side effects add**
3TC 150mg one twice/day beginning on the second week.

After the patient has been on d4T + 3TC for two weeks, send an HIV viral level to determine its effect. As soon as this lab result is available (usually one to two weeks later), review this with the patient, and add it to the T4/HIV graph.

If the HIV viral level has dropped by at least 50% (and preferably 80% to 90%) from the pre-treatment HIV viral level and there are no side effects, then the combination is safe and effective. Proceed to add **Nelfinavir 250mg - three capsules three times per day** (an alternative is Crixivan 400mg - two capsules three times per day).

After one month on d4T + 3TC + Nelfinavir (or Crixivan), have the patient redo the T cell panel, HIV viral level, and chemistry, review them with the patient, and add these labs to the T4/HIV graph [*see Figure 10*]. By that time, the HIV viral level should be undetectable, and the T4 count should be starting to rise. If no side effects, continue therapy. Follow up labs and doctor-patient visits should be done every two to three months to insure no problems have developed and that the patient is maintained in Remission. If any significant side effects, switch to a different triple therapy [*see Figure 6*].

Note that AZT + 3TC + Nelfinavir (or Crixivan) may be used instead of d4T + 3TC + Nelfinavir (or Crixivan), as they are all effective. Many prefer d4T over AZT as the side effect rate with AZT is 30% and only 10% with d4T.

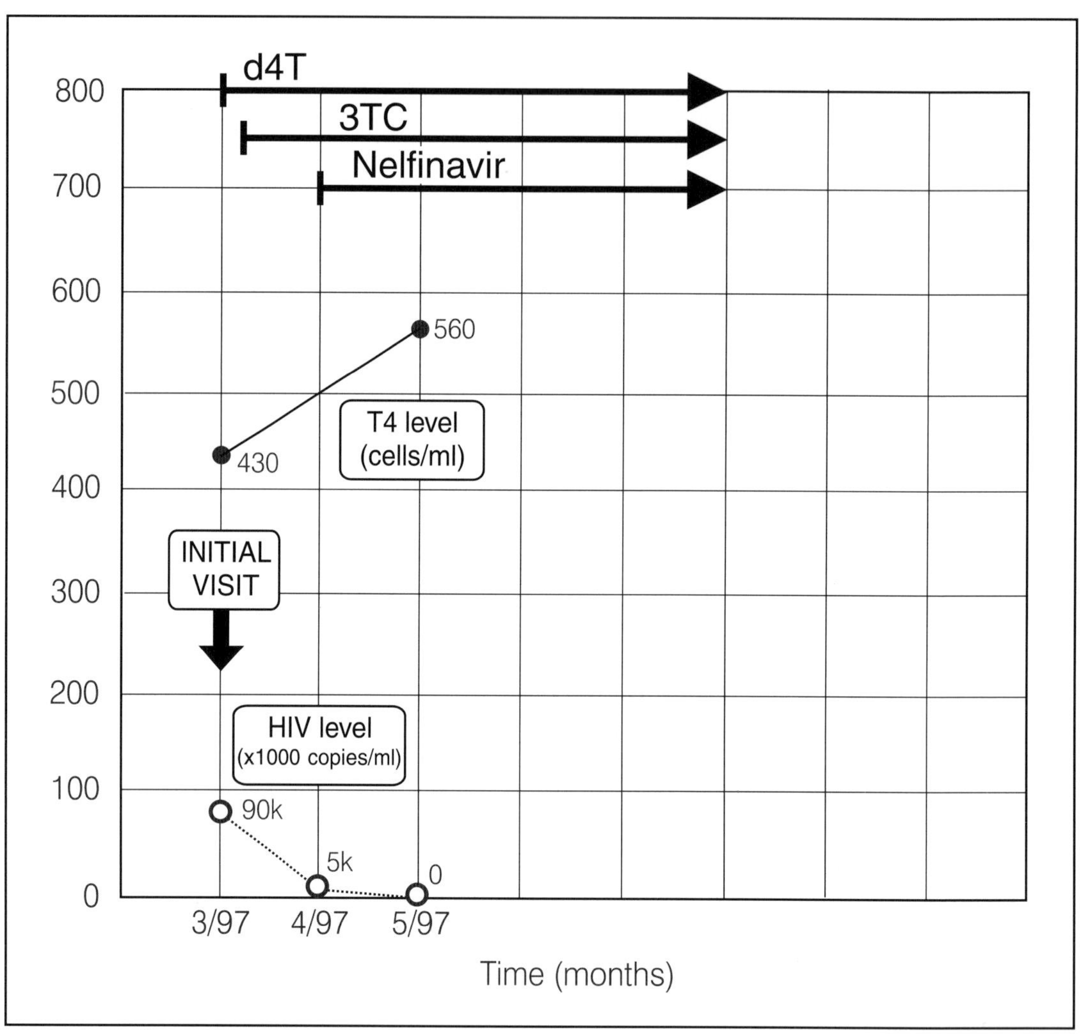

Figure 10 **The T4/HIV graph for this new patient starting triple therapy shows an initial T4 count of 430 rising to 560, and an initial HIV viral level of 90,000 decreasing to 5,000 after therapy with d4T + 3TC, then dropping to zero after the addition of the Protease Inhibitor Nelfinavir.**

Many patients have had prior therapy for HIV infection and a second recipe is useful for starting triple therapy in these cases [*see Figure 11*].

Figure 11 **A recipe for beginning triple therapy in a person with <u>prior</u> therapy.**

You will need:

d4T <u>or</u> AZT

3TC <u>or</u> ddI

Nelfinavir <u>or</u> Crixivan

a good lab with an HIV PCR sensitive to 20 copies/ml

On initial visit, complete a full physical exam including current symptoms, past medical history, allergies, current medicines, vaccination history, places lived, job type, exposure to Tuberculosis, vital signs, and weight. In addition, since the patient has had prior treatment, graph all previous HIV medicines taken, previous T4 cell counts, and HIV viral levels on the patient's T4/HIV graph [*see Figure 12*].

Send labs for T cell panel, HIV Quantitative RNA PCR, Chem 20, CBC/ diff, RPR, Hep A, B, C serologies, and Toxoplasma IgG. If an HIV Resistance Assay is available, this test would be useful to identify resistant patterns. If the patient has had any exposure to TB, place a TB skin test and read it in two days. On return visit in two weeks, the review the lab results with the patient. The T4 cell count and HIV viral level (RNA PCR) are graphed onto the patient's T4/HIV graph with the patient's previous T4 counts and HIV viral levels [*see Figure 12*].

If the patient came to the doctor on **single therapy AZT** for more than six months, then he or she are likely resistant to AZT. Change to d4T for two weeks, do an HIV viral level, and then add 3TC, repeating the labs of an HIV viral level two weeks after the patient is on the d4T + 3TC combination. If the HIV viral level has dropped by 50% or more then add the Protease Inhibitor Crixivan at 800mg three times per day (Nelfinavir at 750mg three times per day is an equally good alternative).

If the person comes to you on **single therapy d4T** for more than six months, he or she may be resistant to d4T. If the HIV viral level is less than 30,000, and especially less than 10,000, add 3TC and recheck the HIV viral level in two weeks. An alternative is to change the person to AZT if they have never had AZT, redo the viral level in two weeks, then add 3TC and do another viral level two weeks after being on AZT + 3TC. The viral level on AZT alone can be compared to the viral level on d4T. Choose the drug that produces the lower HIV viral level. Then add a Protease Inhibitor, either Crixivan or Nelfinavir, and do follow-up labs in four to eight weeks. By then the patient should be in Remission with an undetectable viral level and a rising T4 level. Follow up labs and visits are every two to three months if no problems occur and Remission is being maintained.

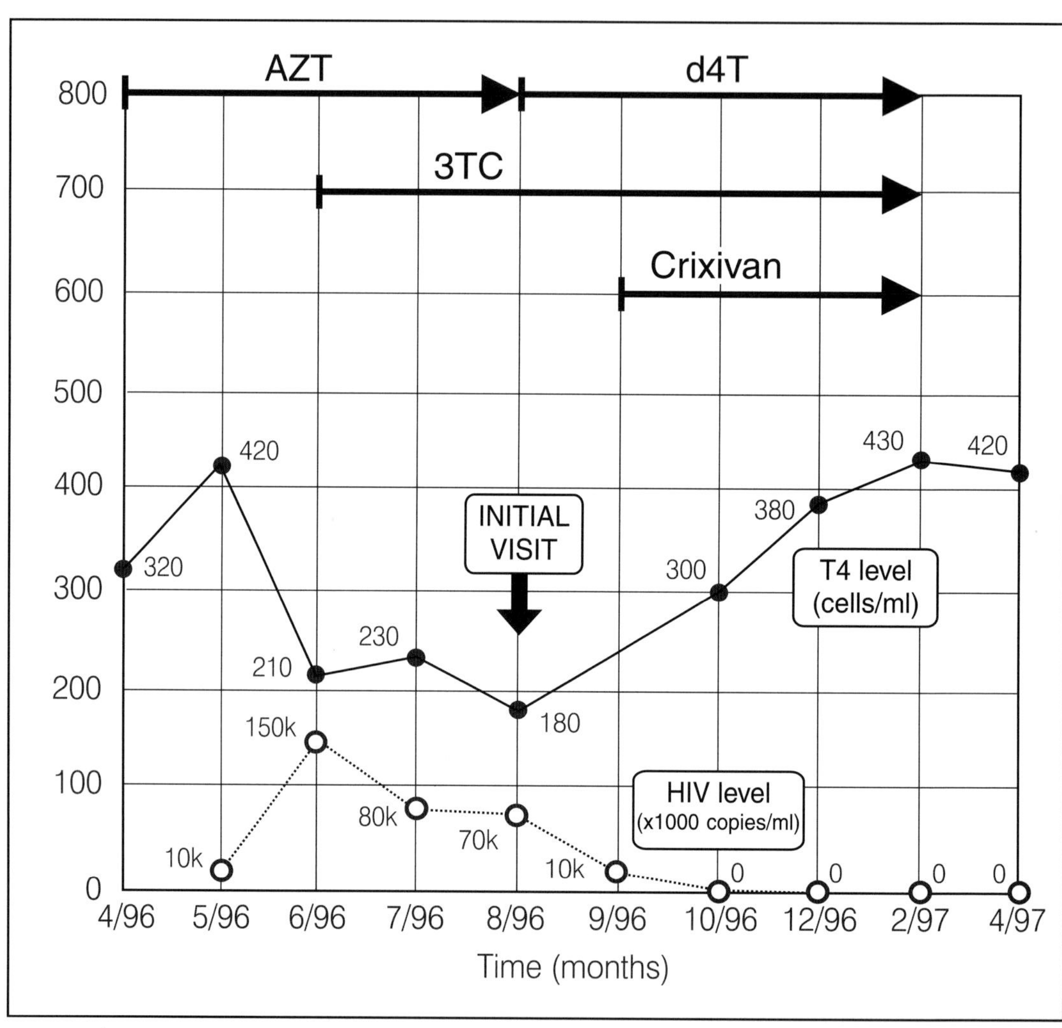

Figure 12 **Changing therapy in a person with prior treatment is challenging. Here the T4/HIV graph shows failing AZT (HIV levels rising from 10,000 to 150,000), good response to 3TC (HIV 150,000 to 70,000), good response to a change to d4T + 3TC (HIV dropping to 10,000), and Remission on d4T + 3TC + Crixivan (HIV level zero and T4 count rising from 180 to 430).**

A third common scenario might be a person who comes to a physician on **either AZT + 3TC *or* d4T + 3TC**. In either case, if the viral level is less than 30,000 and especially less than 10,000, one can safely estimate that the therapy is effective, and go ahead and add a Protease Inhibitor, either Nelfinavir or Crixivan, to complete the triple therapy. If the viral level is greater than 30,000, change from AZT + 3TC to d4T + 3TC, or from d4T + 3TC to AZT + 3TC depending on which one the patient is currently taking. If there are no side effects and the follow-up HIV viral level at two weeks is much lower (50% or more), then go ahead and add Crixivan or Nelfinavir to complete the triple therapy.

If one suspects resistance, or if the pre-treatment therapy is complex and ineffective, then go to Chapter 6, which describes how to analyze and resolve complex cases that may involve multi-resistant HIV infection.

TRIPLE THERAPY WORKS

Using one of four triple therapies, d4T/3TC/Crixivan, AZT/3TC/Crixivan, d4T/3TC/Nelfinavir, or AZT/3TC/Nelfinavir, I have been able to effectively treat 95% of patients who have never received therapy and 80% of those who have had previous therapy. All these therapies are exceedingly effective and easily reduce HIV viral levels to zero within four to eight weeks and usually sooner. I prefer to start with d4T/3TC/Nelfinavir or d4T/3TC/Crixivan, as recent data has shown d4T/3TC to be as good or slightly more effective than AZT/3TC, and d4T/3TC is tolerated in more than 90% of patients (versus 70% in AZT/3TC). Both Protease Inhibitors, Nelfinavir and Crixivan, are extremely effective and easily tolerated, although Nelfinavir is more convenient to take and a bit safer than Crixivan.

As with any medical condition, there are occasionally cases that do not fit the norm. In the case of HIV infection, almost all of these abnormal cases are among those patients who have been on single therapy or prolonged combination therapy and who are resistant to one or more of their medicines. There are rare cases where a patient has side effects to AZT and also d4T. In such cases, I move to alternative triple therapies and determine sensitivity or resistance to each medication using Comparison PCR. This is described in detail in Chapter 6.

The simple global HIV treatment guideline is: **Treat all people with HIV infection at all levels with aggressive triple therapy. Do whatever is necessary to attain an HIV viral level of zero and keep it at zero.** The most successful, simple, and safe therapies are d4T/3TC/Crixivan, AZT/3TC/Crixivan, d4T/3TC/Nelfinavir, and AZT/3TC/Nelfinavir. With these triple therapies, almost all cases of HIV infection can be quickly and effectively treated and placed in Remission.

6
VIRAL RESISTANCE:
Identification & Treatment

6 VIRAL RESISTANCE:
Identification & Treatment

HIV MAKES 10 MILLION CHANGES PER DAY

Resistance in HIV is the formation of an HIV strain that no longer is suppressed by a given medicine or therapy. HIV is one of the most changing or mutagenic infections ever discovered in humans, making replication "errors" at an estimated rate of 10 million mutations a day in every infected person. It does this by randomly altering its genetic code, thus producing differences in most of its structure, including its outer coat, core proteins, reverse transcriptase, protease, integrase, and receptors.

The impact of HIV's ability to mutate cannot be overemphasized. If HIV was unable to change and remained stable, the human immune system would likely shut it down during initial infection. If HIV could not mutate, it probably would be no more serious than the common cold, or at worst, chickenpox or mononucleosis. AIDS as we know it today would not exist.

Untreated, or poorly treated by single or combination therapy, HIV continues to replicate and produce mutations, which produce resistant HIV strains, which break through the attacks of the immune system and medicines, which increase HIV viral levels, which damage the immune system, which decreases T4 cell levels, which makes the person vulnerable to infections, which results in AIDS and finally, death.

TREATING MUTATING INFECTIONS

In most mutating infections, such as Pseudomonas bacteria or Tuberculosis bacteria for example, we send a sample of the infected fluid to the lab for sensitivity testing. What comes back is the name and identification of the particular strain or type of infection, and its sensitivity pattern, a list of all medicines that may possibly be used to treat the infection, and whether they will work or not for this exact specimen [*see Figure 1*]. Then doctor and patient choose a combination of sensitive or effective medicines to treat the infection.

Figure 1 **A Sensitivity Assay lists those medicines that are effective (sensitive) and those that will not work (resistant) for a given infection.**

Name: John Doe **Date of Sample:** 03-01-97

Sample Type: Blood

Isolate Found: **Pseudomonas aeruginosa (bacteria)**

R - Aztreonam
S - Amikacin
S - Ciprofloxacin
R - Ceftazidime
S - Gentamicin
S - Tobramycin
R - Ceftriaxone

S = sensitive (the medicine is effective for this isolate)
R = resistant (the medicine does not significantly suppress growth of this isolate)

In the case of Pseudomonas aeruginosa bacteria, the doctor would order two or three of the sensitive medicines to be taken simultaneously. From historical studies, it is clear that for Pseudomonas, two sensitive medicines are effective treatment. If a particular infection mutates more rapidly, such as with HIV infection, three sensitive medicines administered simultaneously will be necessary to shut off the infection.

SENSITIVE, VARIABLE, & COMPLETE RESISTANCE

If a medicine easily and heavily suppresses replication of a particular HIV strain, dropping the HIV viral level by at least 50%, and usually by 90% within two weeks, this HIV strain is **sensitive** to this medicine. If a medicine only slightly or partially suppresses replication of a particular HIV strain (to, say, 30%), the HIV strain has **variable resistance** to the medicine tested. In some cases of variable resistance, the virus may be more fully suppressed by increasing the dose of the medicine. If a medicine has no effect on the replication of a particular HIV strain, that HIV strain has **complete resistance** to the medicine [*see Figure 2*].

WE NEED AN ACCURATE HIV SENSITIVITY ASSAY

At this writing, there is no accurate HIV Sensitivity Assay commercially available, although there are some labs in the United States and Europe who are performing these tests on a very limited basis. Recently an HIV Genotype or gene sequencing assay became available at some labs. This assay only samples a limited number of HIV, providing useful information on their gene patterns. However, there is a mixture of different HIV strains in each person. The results might represent the overall pattern of HIV in a person or they might represent an insignificant HIV strain typical of a tiny percent of that person's HIV infection. There is no way to tell, making the HIV Genotype test difficult to interpret or use.

Currently there is no other test more needed than an accurate and widely available HIV Sensitivity Assay. With it, doctors would be able to have their patient's blood drawn and analyzed once or twice a year. The HIV Sensitivity Assay results would enable the doctor to choose or verify that all three medicines of the prescribed triple therapy were sensitive, meaning that the patient's current strain of HIV was being shut off by each of the three medicines individually.

Currently, most doctors do the best they can by simply guessing, and even among the most experienced of us, our guesses are probably 50% accurate at best, more likely no better than 30% accurate. If it is the case that one or two medicines in a triple therapy are resistant (ineffective), the patient may as well be on a two drug or one drug therapy [*see Figure 3*]. And as we now know, either of these will fail in a fairly short period of time. It is absolutely critical for the successful treatment of HIV infection that all three medicines in the triple therapy are working. Resistance is common in complex cases, especially those with:

- prior prolonged single therapy,
- prior prolonged double therapy with dropping T4 and/or rising HIV PCR,
- cases that were failing, where medicines were slowly added one at a time over one to two years (i.e. AZT then 3TC then Crixivan),
- cases with high viral levels on therapy (PCR greater than 30,000 or so).

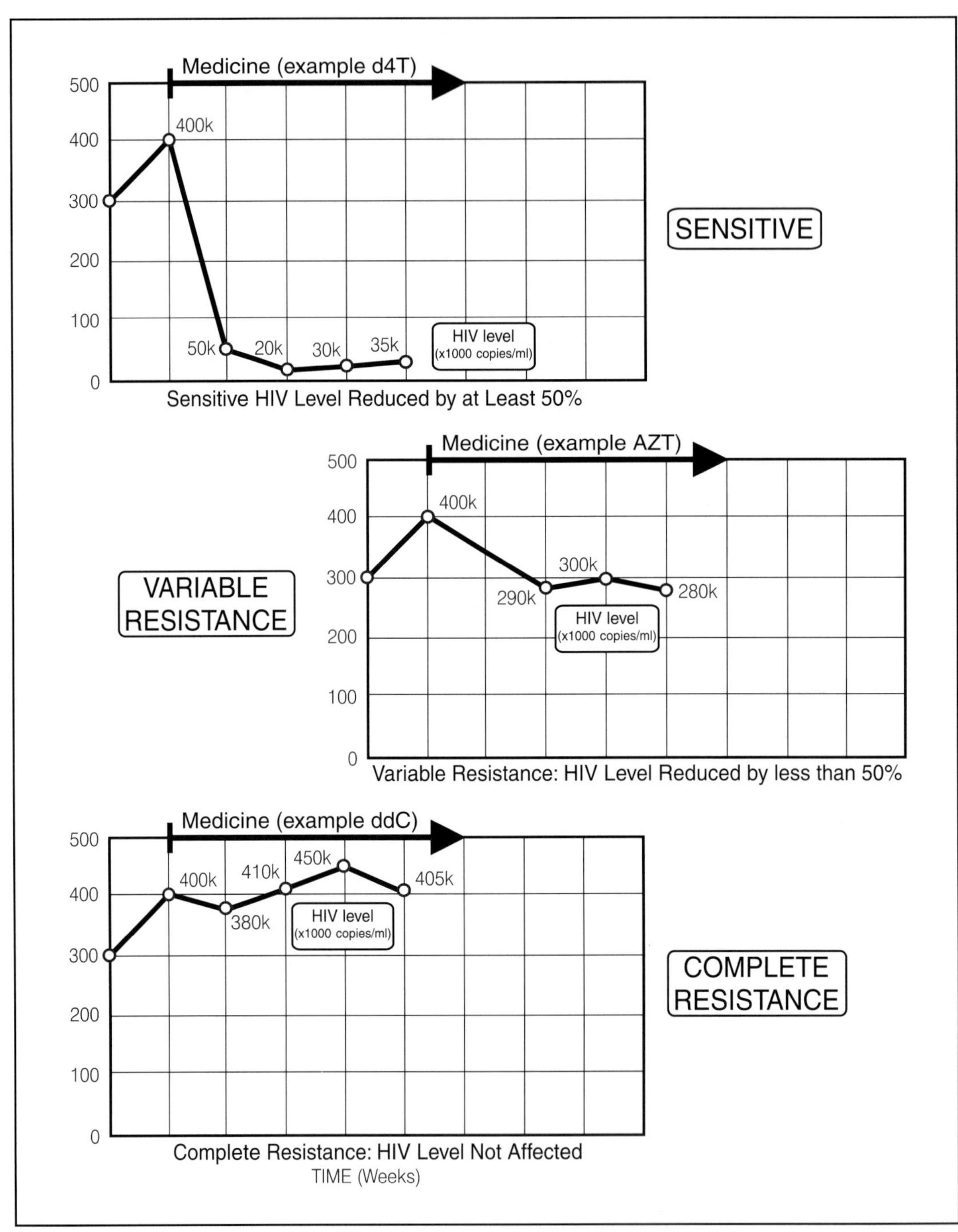

Figure 2 **HIV may be sensitive, or have variable or complete resistance to a particular medicine. If sensitive, the HIV level drops by more than 50% when the medicine is added. In complete resistance, the HIV level does not significantly change, and in variable resistance the HIV level change is less than a 50%.**

Resistance is unlikely to exist, and therefore resistance testing is not essential when:

- treatment is being initiated for the first time (but remember to check the PCR and make sure HIV viral levels are rapidly dropping after adding the first or second medicine),
- those cases with zero or very low viral levels (PCR less than 10,000) who never were on prolonged single therapy.

Figure 3 **Errors in Choosing Triple Therapy and Their Results**

If a person is on:

Drug A	**(sensitive)**		
+			
Drug B	**(sensitive)**	**= Triple therapy**	**= Treatment success**
+			
Drug C	**(sensitive)**		

If a person is on:

Drug A	**(resistant)**		
+			
Drug B	**(sensitive)**	**= Double therapy**	**= Limited effectiveness**
+			
Drug C	**(sensitive)**		

If a person is on:

Drug A	**(resistant)**		
+			
Drug B	**(resistant)**	**= Single therapy**	**= Failure**
+			
Drug C	**(sensitive)**		

If a person is on:

Drug A	**(resistant)**		
+			
Drug B	**(resistant)**	**= No therapy**	**= Failure**
+			
Drug C	**(resistant)**		

Without an HIV Sensitivity Assay, how do you insure effective triple therapy? You can evaluate whether a medicine is sensitive by making a **Comparison HIV Viral Level**, comparing the initial baseline HIV viral level with a second HIV viral level after two weeks of therapy on the medicine in question. It's what I use until an accurate HIV Sensitivity Assay becomes available. If the technique used is HIV viral level by Quantitative RNA PCR, I call it **Comparison PCR** [*see Figure 4*].

Figure 4 **To determine if a medicine is effective, compare pre and post treatment PCRs. I call this Comparison PCR.**

Comparison PCR is done as follows:

1. Draw an HIV Quantitative RNA PCR. At this PCR, the person would be on no HIV medicines, or would have been on the same therapy for a minimum of two weeks.

2. Add the medicine of interest.

3. Draw a second HIV Quantitative RNA PCR after the patient has been taking the medicine for two weeks.

4. Evaluate the results as follows:

Sensitive: 50% or more decrease in PCR.

Resistant: No decrease in PCR, or a drop of less than 50%.

*Note, in determining how useful an HIV medicine is, I only evaluate results as sensitive or resistant. I don't believe this technique is accurate enough to determine variable resistance.

In planning effective triple therapy for people with HIV infection, be as sure as possible that every medicine you use is sensitive, and therefore effective and useful in each case.

Remember, HIV medicines have one job: to lower HIV viral level. If they don't do this for the patient, they are not useful, should be thrown out, and other medicines substituted. Also, keep in mind that if a person has an HIV infection that is resistant to a particular medicine or medicines, this resistant pattern is likely to last for the rest of that person's life. The medicine should be marked as permanently resistant on the individual's chart.

EXAMPLE CASES

Case 1: HIV Previously Untreated

Data: A 30-year-old man, HIV positive for at least six years, has never taken any HIV medicines. He decides that he wants to give treatment a try and asks for your help. His T4 count five years ago was 800, declining to 380 one month ago. Labs are done today revealing a T4 - 368, HIV Quantitative RNA PCR - 112,000, and blood counts and chemistry - normal. You create a T4/PCR graph of his data [*see Figure 5*].

Comment: Never having taken HIV medicines, he has "wild type" HIV, the most common HIV strain in those infected, which is usually sensitive to all medicines. It is probably not necessary to check every medicine of the triple therapy individually, although this could be done to be absolutely sure. I recommend checking the PCR after this man is successfully on two drug therapy, then, if that's working well, add a Protease Inhibitor as a third medicine. Then check the T4 count and PCR (HIV viral level) again after he has been on the triple therapy for two to four weeks.

Treatment: Instruct the patient to start AZT 300mg - one twice per day (d4T at 40mg twice per day would be just as good). After one week, when his minor nausea has resolved, add 3TC at 150mg one twice per day to the AZT.

After two weeks on AZT + 3TC, the HIV Quantitative RNA PCR (HIV viral level) is 5000 copies of HIV RNA/ml. Crixivan at 400mg - two capsules taken three times per day is added to complete the triple therapy (Nelfinavir is an equally good alternative to Crixivan).

After an additional two to four weeks of therapy, labs are redrawn with normal blood counts (the red cell mean cell volume, MCV, is mildly elevated due to AZT but this causes no harm), normal chemistry, T4 - 510, and PCR less than 20 (undetectable) [*seen graphically in Figure 5*]. After an additional three months on therapy, the T4 count rises to 750, while the HIV level remains zero.

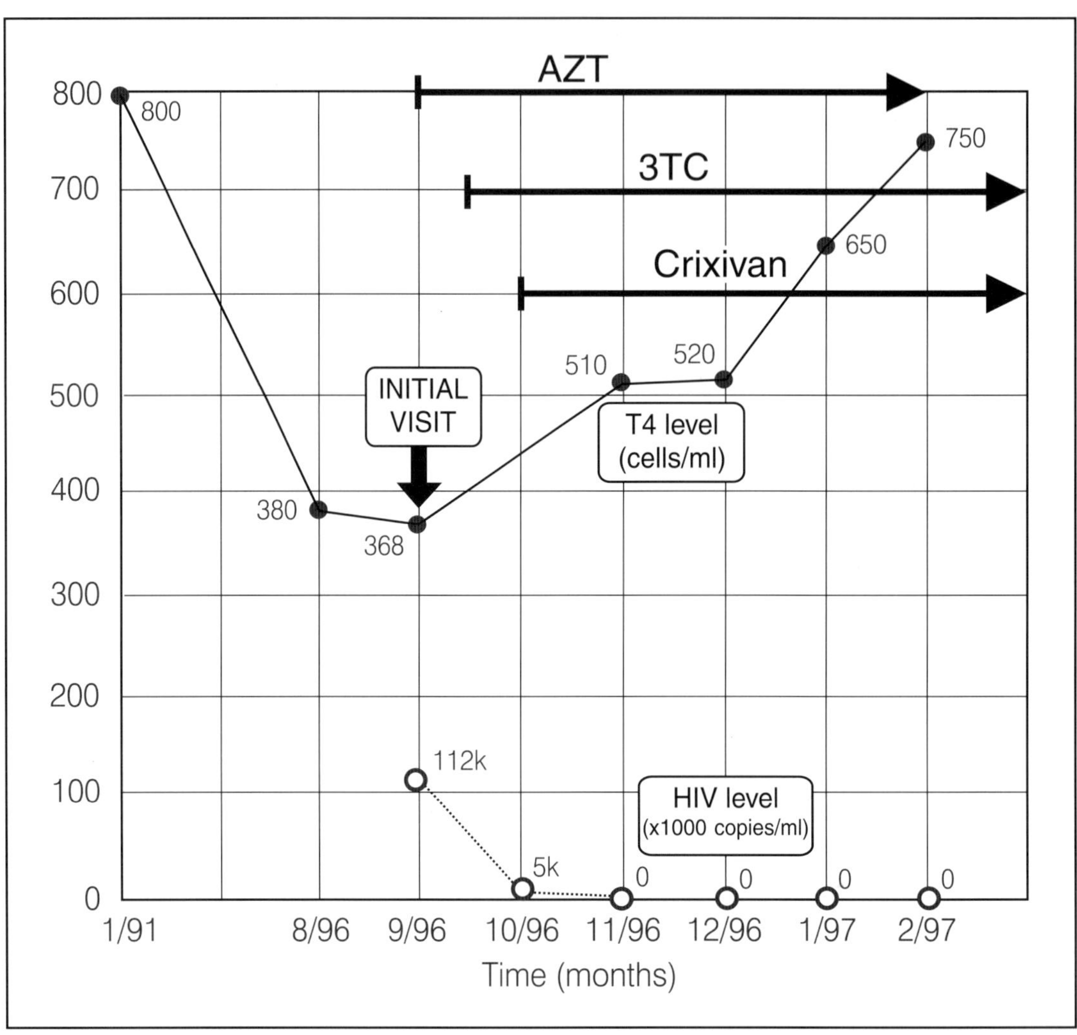

Figure 5 **The T4/HIV graph for Case 1, previously untreated: the HIV level decreases from 112,000 to 5,000 on AZT + 3TC, and to zero on AZT + 3TC + Crixivan. The T4 count in response increases from 368 to 510 and later to 750.**

This is excellent therapy for the patient. He is now in Remission without side effects, and with an immune system that is gaining strength. The conclusion of the Comparison PCR is that this person is **sensitive to AZT + 3TC** and **sensitive to Crixivan**. I would assume he is individually **sensitive to AZT** and **sensitive to 3TC**.

Case 2: HIV Previously Treated with AZT & ddI as Single Therapy

Data: A 40-year-old woman was previously on AZT single therapy for four years with declining T4 levels. She was changed by her previous doctor to ddI with a temporary increase in T4 count which is now again dropping. She comes to you for help, since you are known to solve difficult cases. Her T4 count six months ago on ddI was 280 with an HIV Quantitative RNA PCR then of 28,000. Labs are redrawn today showing T4 - 130 and PCR - 75,000. Blood counts and chemistry are normal. You graph her data on a T4/HIV graph [*see Figure 6*].

Comment: She likely is resistant to AZT due to her prolonged AZT single therapy and her dropping T4 count while on AZT therapy. She is resistant to ddI demonstrated by a rising HIV PCR (28,000 increasing to 75,000), and confirmed by a dropping T4. No further testing of AZT or ddI is necessary given the history. This is a typical case of a well intentioned doctor who followed bad guidelines, ruining the chances of two good medicines ever helping this woman.

Treatment: Due to single therapy in the past, which almost always produces this bad result, you realize the patient has a multi-resistant HIV strain . You stop her ddI, and tell her not to take AZT. Next you start her on d4T at 40mg, one twice each day.

After two weeks of d4T, you check a PCR, and tell her to add 3TC at 150mg, one twice per day. After two more weeks of the d4T + 3TC, you have her redo her T4 count, HIV PCR, and chemistry. Note that, rarely, d4T may cross resist with AZT, and 3TC may cross resist with ddI; lets hope not here.

After two weeks of d4T, her HIV PCR has dropped from 75,000 to 15,000. After two weeks of d4T + 3TC, her PCR has dropped further to 3,000, and her T4 is 200. You graph these labs on her T4/HIV graph [*see Figure 6*] and then have her add Crixivan at 400mg, two capsules three time per day (Nelfinavir is an equally good alternative).

After four weeks of d4T + 3TC + Crixivan, her PCR is 500, her T4 is 270, and her chemistry is normal. After two months of d4T + 3TC + Crixivan, her PCR is undetectable (less than 20), and her T4 is 340. Graph these again on her T4/HIV graph [*see Figure 6*].

Conclusion: The patient tells you that she has not felt this good in more than four years. She is **resistant to AZT**, **resistant to ddI**, **sensitive to d4T**, **sensitive to 3TC**, and **sensitive to Crixivan.**

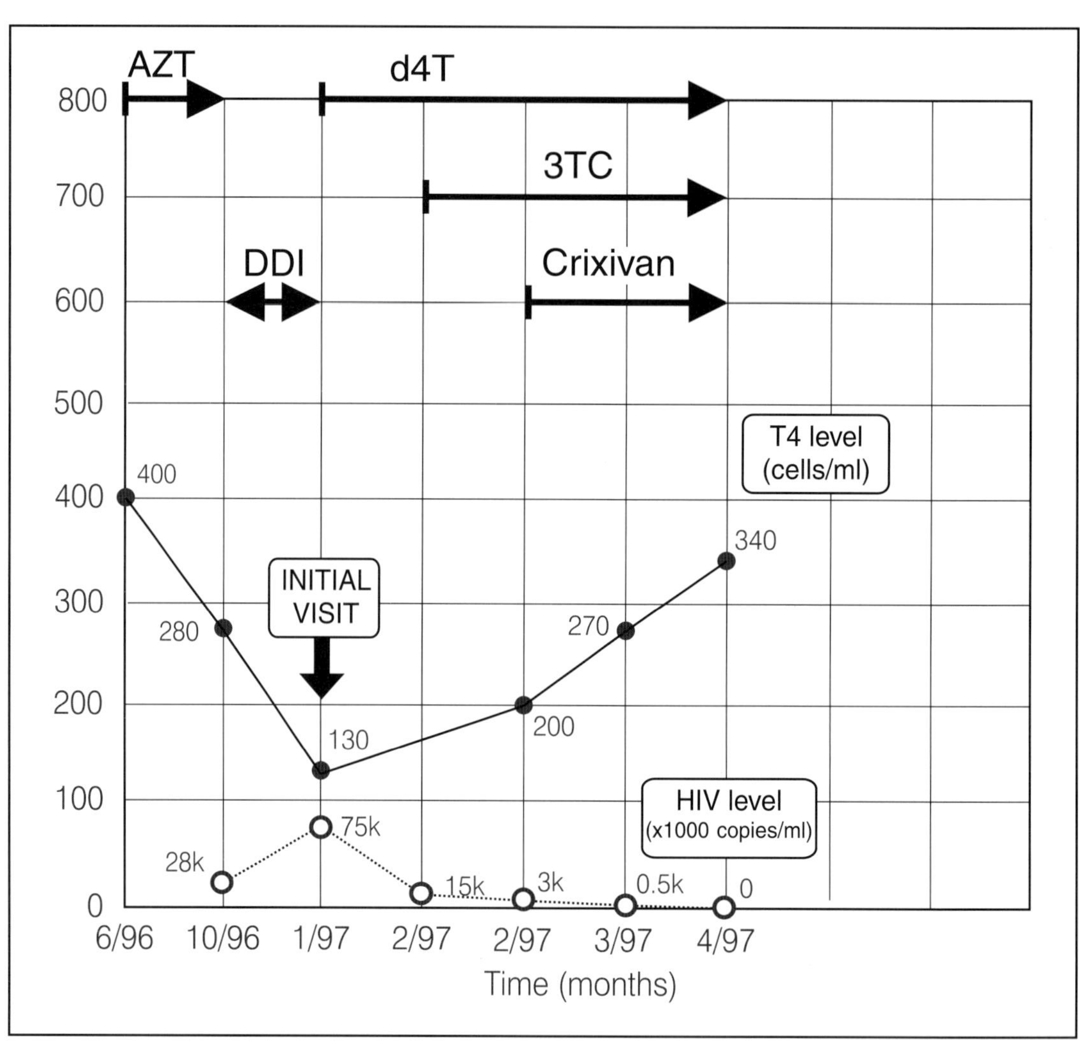

Figure 6 **The T4/HIV graph for Case 2: previously treated with AZT & ddI. AZT fails with a T4 count decrease from 400 to 280. ddI fails with a dropping T4 count and a rising HIV viral level (28,000 to 75,000). d4T is successful with the HIV level dropping from 75,000 to 15,000, as does 3TC (HIV-15,000 to 3,000). Remission is achieved with the addition of Crixivan and the T4 count rises to 340.**

Case 3: HIV Previously Treated with Multiple HIV Medicines

Data: A 35-year-old man asks for your help. He has had five years of multiple drug therapy, including single therapy AZT, AZT + ddC, ddI, AZT + ddI, AZT + 3TC, and more recently AZT + 3TC + Saquinavir, and AZT + 3TC + Ritonavir. He has had numbness and pain (neuropathy) in his feet while taking d4T and does not want to try it again. He has had severe nausea, vomiting, and malaise since beginning Ritonavir six weeks ago. Three months ago, on AZT + 3TC, his T4 was 30 and his viral level was 120,000. Six weeks ago, his T4 was 90 and his PCR was 110,000 on AZT + 3TC + Saquinavir. His current T4 is 150 with a viral level of 54,000 on AZT + 3TC + Ritonavir, although he admits missing "a lot" of doses of his medicines due to his nausea and vomiting. You graph his data on a T4/HIV graph [*see Figure 7*].

Comment: Having taken so many medicines in different combinations, it is truly unclear what is working here. His recent therapy of AZT + 3TC + Saquinavir did not reduce HIV significantly (HIV PCR 120,000 to 110,000). The AZT + 3TC + Ritonavir therapy was somewhat more effective, given his decreasing PCRs (110,000 to 54,000) and his rising T4 (90 to 150). However, the issue of new Protease Inhibitor (Ritonavir) resistance arises due to his missed doses. Additionally, he is feeling terrible since beginning Ritonavir.

Treatment: He is quite ill with nausea and vomiting. You instruct him to **stop AZT, stop 3TC, and stop Ritonavir.** To your relief, a blood count, chemistry, and amylase (pancreas test) are normal. He is back to good health and a full diet in five days. After two weeks **off** AZT, 3TC, and Ritonavir, you have him draw an HIV Quantitative RNA PCR, and then begin the AZT at 300mg, one twice per day. After two weeks of AZT, he still feels fine and does a second PCR. After this second PCR, he advances his therapy to AZT + 3TC with 3TC at 150mg, one twice per day. After two more weeks of AZT + 3TC he has a T4 and PCR drawn and sent.

You see him to review these results. His baseline PCR off all therapy is 740,000. After two weeks of AZT, his PCR drops to 300,000. After two more weeks of AZT + 3TC, his PCR is 90,000 and his T4 is 120. You tell him that fortunately both AZT and 3TC are sensitive. You complete his therapy by having him add Crixivan at 400mg, two three times per day. After one month of AZT + 3TC + Crixivan, his PCR is 2,000 and his T4 is 230. After two months of AZT + 3TC + Crixivan, his PCR is 600 and his T4 is 320. At three months his PCR is undetectable (less than 20), and his T4 is 380 [*see Figure 7*].

Conclusion: sensitive to AZT, sensitive to 3TC, sensitive to Crixivan, sensitive to Ritonavir (although intolerable side effects in this case), and **resistant to Saquinavir** (PCR 120,000 to 110,000, which is less than a 50% drop).

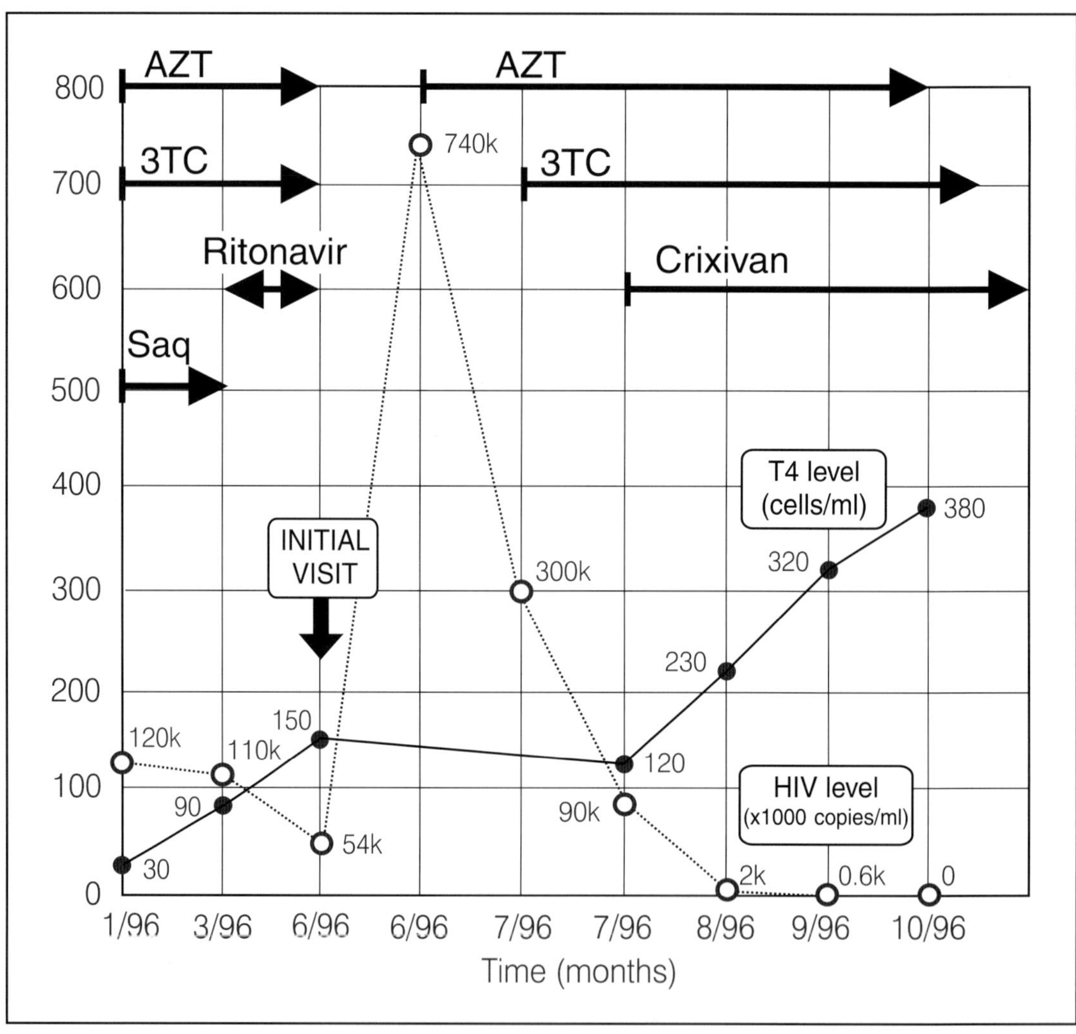

Figure 7 **The T4/HIV graph for Case 3: HIV with multiple prior therapies. Sometimes it is necessary to temporarily stop therapy. Here the HIV level rises to 740,000, drops to 300,000 on AZT, to 90,000 after 3TC is added, and to 2,000 and then to zero after Crixivan is added. The T4 count rises from 150 to 380.**

Case 4: Why Not Just Add a Protease Inhibitor?

Data: A 38-year-old man who was on AZT single therapy for four years had 3TC added to his treatment by his prior doctor six months ago. He comes to you for "protease therapy" as his current doctor did not want to add it, saying "You're stable, and I don't want to waste your options too early." The patient has never had a viral level. His T4 was 450 about four years ago, and in his past two labs six and three months ago, his T4 was 120 and 140, respectively. He was told these drops in T4 are "normal" for someone with HIV. He wants to add a Protease Inhibitor. You have him do labs which reveal a T4 of 130, and an HIV Quantitative RNA PCR of 90,000. You graph his data on a T4/HIV graph [*see Figure 8*].

Comment: Does he have serial resistance due to single use AZT and the addition of 3TC, or are AZT and/or 3TC working? Since it is unclear, you decide to get an HIV Quantitative RNA PCR while he is off treatment, and analyze his treatment by Comparison PCR.

Treatment: You convince him to stop AZT and stop 3TC for two weeks, and then redo his PCR. Using an instruction sheet you write for him, he restarts the AZT after the lab is drawn, waits two more weeks on AZT, and repeats the PCR while on AZT. After the second PCR, he adds 3TC at 150mg one twice per day to his AZT, 100mg, two twice per day. By that time his labs have come in.

His viral level off therapy is 100,000. On AZT alone, it is 105,000 with a T4 count of 145. You conclude that neither AZT nor 3TC are working as there has been no significant difference on his PCRs from AZT + 3TC (90,000), no therapy (100,000), and AZT (105,000). You graph these results on his T4/HIV graph and tell him that, unfortunately neither AZT nor 3TC are of any benefit to him, and tell him to stop both of them for good this time. Next you start him on d4T 40mg, one twice per day for two weeks and then have him do another PCR. Then you have him add ddI 100mg, two twice per day on an empty stomach, so that now he is on d4T + ddI. After two weeks on this new therapy, you repeat his PCR and T4 level.

His labs show a PCR of 15,000 after two weeks of d4T single therapy. After two weeks of d4T + ddI, his PCR is undetectable (less than 20) and his T4 count rises to 360. Finally to complete the triple therapy, the patient adds the Protease Inhibitor Crixivan, 400mg, at two capsules taken three times per day (Nelfinavir is an equally good alternative). After two months on Crixivan + d4T + ddI, this man's HIV viral level remains undetectable, and his T4 level has risen to 540 [*see Figure 8*].

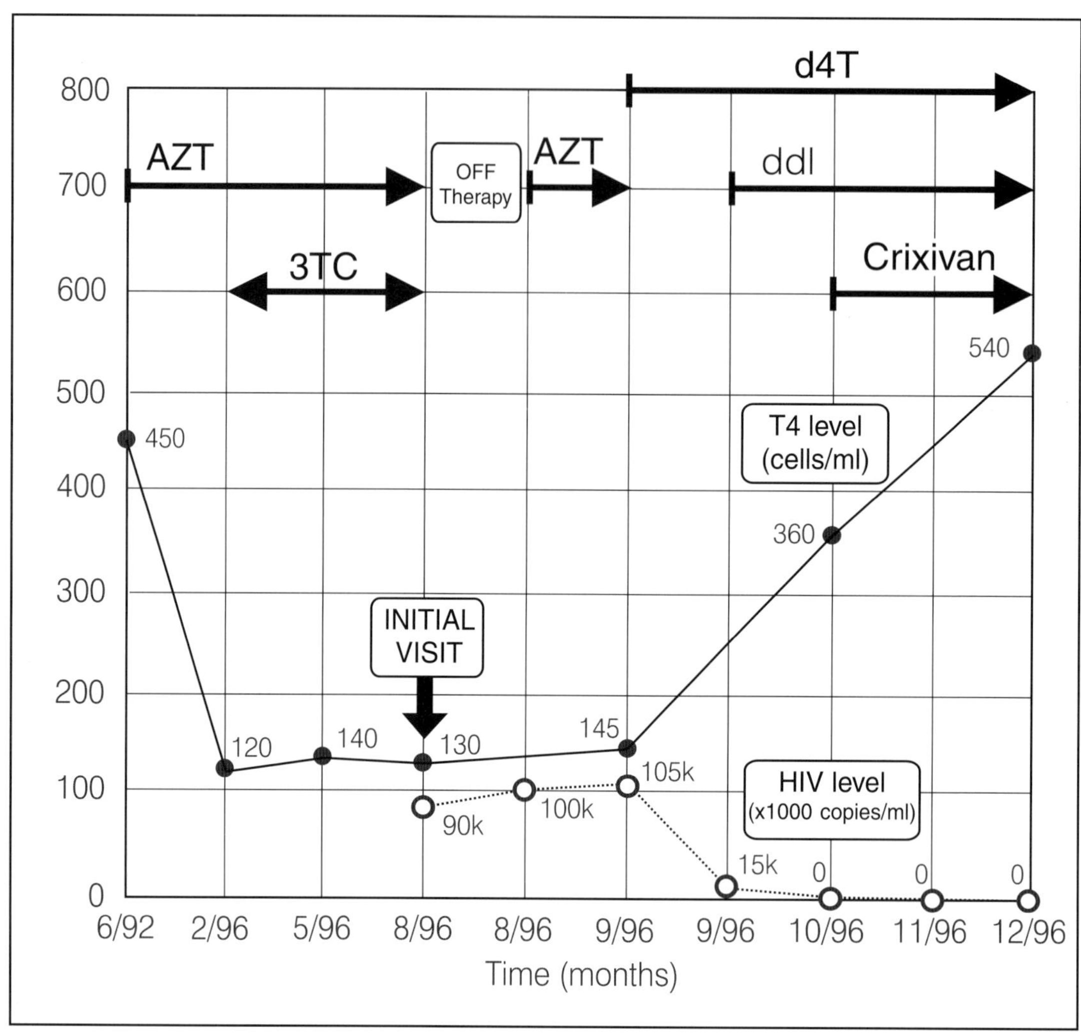

Figure 8 **The T4/HIV graph for Case 4: Why not just add a Protease Inhibitor? Off therapy the HIV level is almost the same as on AZT + 3TC showing that they were having no effect. With d4T, the HIV level drops from 105,000 to 15,000, and to zero and remains at zero with the addition of ddI and Crixivan. The T4 count rises from 145 to 540.**

Conclusion: resistant-AZT, resistant-3TC, sensitive-d4T, sensitive-ddI, sensitive-Crixivan. This is a classic case of serial resistance, which national guidelines have encouraged doctors and patients to make. Had you or this man's previous doctor added Crixivan to the resistant AZT + 3TC, his therapy would have failed completely in three to six months, and the patient would have been fully and permanently resistant to Crixivan, Ritonavir, and possibly Saquinavir. Effective triple therapy has surely changed his life and could very well be beneficial to him indefinitely.

This is a difficult regimen as ddI must be taken on an empty stomach, and Crixivan cannot be taken within 1 hour of the ddI, or its effectiveness will be greatly reduced. However Crixivan is fine with most carbohydrates. You suggest the following timetable:

Time of Day:	Take:
early AM	ddI
light breakfast	Crixivan + d4T
3pm	Crixivan
4pm	ddI
bedtime	Crixivan + d4T

SOME TIPS FOR DIFFICULT CASES

- Get a full history of prior treatment and all prior T4 and HIV PCR data.
- Always graph the T4 count and HIV PCR, and overlay these graphs with the medicines that were being taken at the time.
- Have a graph of the T4 counts and viral levels in every chart and encourage the patient to keep one as well.
- Update the graph every visit when new T4 and PCR data comes in. Do it with the patient. It takes five seconds and is much easier than paging through two or three inches of lab data.
- Do not stop therapy for more than two weeks if at all possible.
- Do not use single therapy for more than two weeks.
- Do not ever use 3TC, Nevirapine, or Delavirdine as single therapy at all, as viral resistance to these medicines can occur in just two weeks. But they may be added as the second or third medicine when bringing a triple therapy on line.
- Do not wait for lab results to add medicines. Look at labs when they come in and adjust therapy as needed.
- Do not assume if at all possible.

THE PATIENT INSTRUCTION SHEET

Because of the stress related to just seeing a doctor, having an exam, and discussing health issues, the average person remembers only 10% of what the doc tor says during an office visit. HIV therapy is complex, involving multiple medicines, lab tests, and visits, especially in the beginning or when changes are being made. And mistakes lead to treatment failure.

To simplify the process and avoid error, give the patient a written plan. For example:

1. Stop AZT and stop 3TC for two weeks, then
2. Have your labs drawn [include a lab slip for T4 and PCR]
3. Start d4T, 40mg, one twice per day for two weeks, then
4. Have a second set of labs drawn [include a lab slip for PCR]
5. Add 3TC, 150mg, one twice per day, to the d4T,
6. After two more weeks of d4T + 3TC, have the third set of labs drawn [include a lab slip for T4, PCR, & Chemistry]
7. Schedule your next appointment in seven to eight weeks. If any problems, see me immediately.

There's no question that it takes work to get each person with HIV on the correct triple therapy. I tell patients that it will be a "busy first eight weeks." But once doctor and patient find the three medicines that work together with no significant side effects, you're both home free. The triple therapies in mathematical modeling and in real life truly work, virtually indefinitely, when the viral level is driven to zero.

SUMMARY

We have demonstrated how to solve some of the most complex cases of HIV infection involving multi-resistant HIV strains. These types of cases are always difficult to solve, but the time devoted typically produces large health benefits to those patients with multi-resistant HIV. HIV can become resistant to any medicine. We can identify HIV resistance by Comparison PCR. This technique is relatively easy if the data is graphed and gathered at two or three week intervals. Effective medicines drop HIV viral levels by a minimum of 50% and the best medicines lower HIV levels by 80% to 90% after two weeks of treatment. Resistant medicines fail to change HIV viral levels at all or very little, and when found should not be used.

An accurate HIV Sensitivity Assay will be invaluable in helping determine which medicines are able to drive the HIV viral level to zero and keep it there. Meanwhile, there is nothing like real world testing. Resistance testing will always be prone to errors, given HIV's ongoing evolution when it is replicating. Check an HIV PCR two to three weeks after changing therapy to verify that viral level is dropping, regardless of the results of a sensitivity assay.

7
PREVENTING INFECTIONS:
It's as easy as 3 - 2 - 1

7 PREVENTING INFECTIONS:
It's as easy as 3 - 2 - 1

THREE PARTS OF HIV TREATMENT

There are three parts to maintaining good health with HIV infection:

- treating HIV infection with triple therapy,
- preventing infections, and
- reversing Wasting Syndrome (weight loss).

All three areas must be addressed in each case of HIV infection in order to maintain normal health. In this chapter we'll discuss how to prevent infections, but first, some background.

Prior to Dr. Louis Pasteur's landmark discovery of life forms that were not visible to the naked eye, it was assumed that disease was caused by bad air or bad spirits. Now we know that many diseases are caused by the entrance of microscopic life forms from the outside environment into the human body. These "diseases" are called infections. They come in four major categories:

- **Protozoa/amebae** - larger complex, mobile life forms,
- **Fungus** - complex, sometimes branching "plant-like" life forms,
- **Bacteria** - smaller, single cell life forms, and
- **Virus** - tiny protein structures containing DNA or RNA.

The key to preventing infections in people with HIV is knowledge. The following information will act as the basis for our treatment strategy:

People with HIV infection are not at risk for all infections. They are only at risk for specific infections, and their risk for each of these infections can be precisely forecast based on their T4 count at any given time. And today we have medicines that can prevent each of these specific infections.

The eight most common infections, also known as "Opportunistic Infections," in persons with HIV are **Herpes, Zoster, PCP, Cryptococcus, Candida, MAI, CMV, and Toxoplasmosis.** All you need to prevent these infections in people with HIV are a few pieces of data:

- their current T4 count, within the past two to three months,
- where they were born, lived, and traveled, and
- their current living situation, job, and pets.

Both patient and doctor should keep a graph of the individual's T4 counts and viral levels. Over several years, this will provide an accurate picture of the T4 count and the overall trend of the immune system. One also refers to the T4 graph to determine the current functioning level of that person's immune system. Its level of function as measured by the T4 count determines whether that person is at risk for a specific infection at any given time.

IT'S AS EASY AS 3 - 2 - 1

People with HIV infection are at risk for the eight Opportunistic Infections but only if their T4 count drops below certain key levels. The lower the T4 count, the greater the risk for more infections. But when the T4 count increases and therefore the strength of the immune system increases, the risk of infections decreases. With this approach, one can prevent the eight major Opportunistic Infections from occurring.

I follow **the Rule of 3 -2 - 1** where:

3 = a T4 count less than 300,

2 = a T4 count less than 200, and

1 = a T4 count less than 100.

The Rule of 3 - 2 - 1 works and is universally easy to remember and use. The Rule of 3 - 2 - 1 predicts risk of the eight major Opportunistic Infections by the current T4 count [*see Figure 1*]. If the T4 count drops below any of the levels (300, 200, 100), that person is now at risk for additional infections and additional steps should be taken to prevent them.

Figure 1 **The Rule of 3 - 2 - 1 predicts risk of infection based on the current T4 count.**

INFECTION RISK AT EACH T4 LEVEL

T4 Level	Infection Risk
All	**Herpes & Zoster**
T4 Levels less than 300	**PCP**
T4 Levels less than 200	**Cryptococcus, Candida**
T4 Levels less than 100	**MAI, CMV, Toxoplasmosis**

A person's current T4 count determines which infections are likely to occur without prevention. This, in turn, determines which prevention medicines he or she should consider taking to keep the infection from occurring. One can also superimpose the risk of Opportunistic Infections on the T4 graph, forming a visual representation of the Rule of 3 - 2 - 1 [*see Figure 2*].

To prevent these infections, medicines are given on a daily basis as additional protection in case a person with HIV encounters an Opportunistic Infection during their daily activities. In a sense a person with HIV becomes part of their own immune system by actively adding additional medicines to their therapy if their own immune system is too weak at a given time to provide the full protection of a normal immune system.

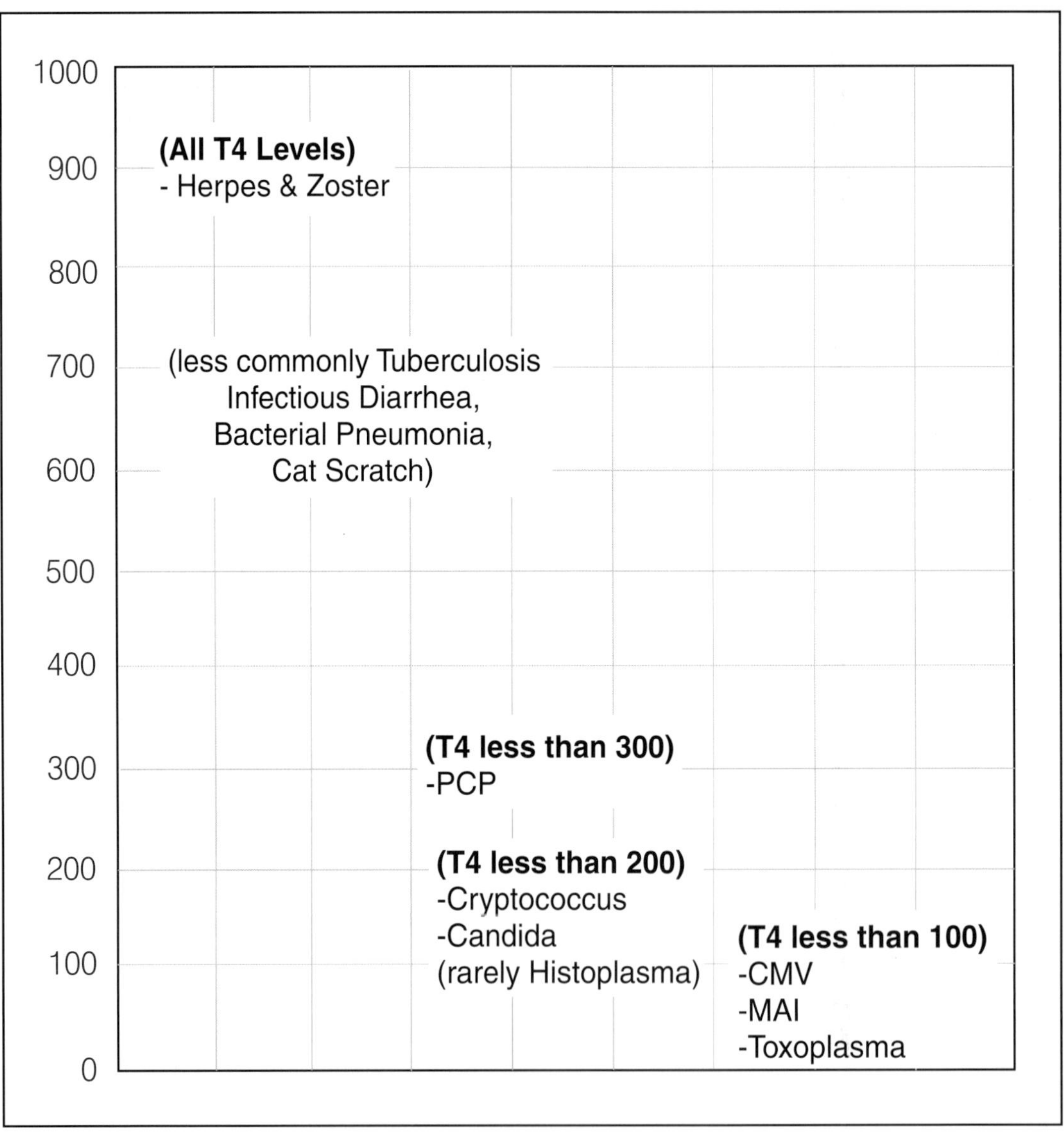

Figure 2 **The Rule of 3 - 2 - 1 determines which Opportunistic Infections occur at differing T4 counts without prevention measures.**

EIGHT INFECTIONS - WHAT THEY ARE & HOW TO PREVENT THEM

Based on our knowledge of risk of infection at each T4 cell level, *Figure 3* lists the medications to take at each T4 level to prevent infections in a person with HIV disease. If properly applied, almost all people with HIV will avoid these Opportunistic Infections during their lifetime.

Medications to Prevent Opportunistic Infections in HIV

T4 Level	At Risk for:	Medication to Take to Prevent the Infection
All	**Herpes/Zoster**	**Acyclovir** 400mg twice per day
less than 300	**PCP**	**Septra** ds or **Dapsone** 100mg/day
less than 200	**Cryptococcus & Candida**	**Fluconazole** 100mg one/day
less than 100	**MAI**	**Biaxin** 500mg twice/day (or Azithromycin 1200mg/week)
	CMV	If **urine or blood +**, then **Cytovene** 1 gram three times/day
	Toxoplasma	If **blood +**, then **Septra** ds one/day, (or **Azithromycin** 250mg twice/day)

Figure 3 **Certain medicines should be added to a person's therapy based on his or her current T4 count. If the T4 count decreases, more medicines are needed to prevent certain Opportunistic Infections. If the T4 count rises, less prevention medicines are required.**

We can overlay the prevention medicines on the T4 graph to create a visual representation of Rule 3 - 2 - 1 as these medicines apply to each T4 level [*see Figure 4*].

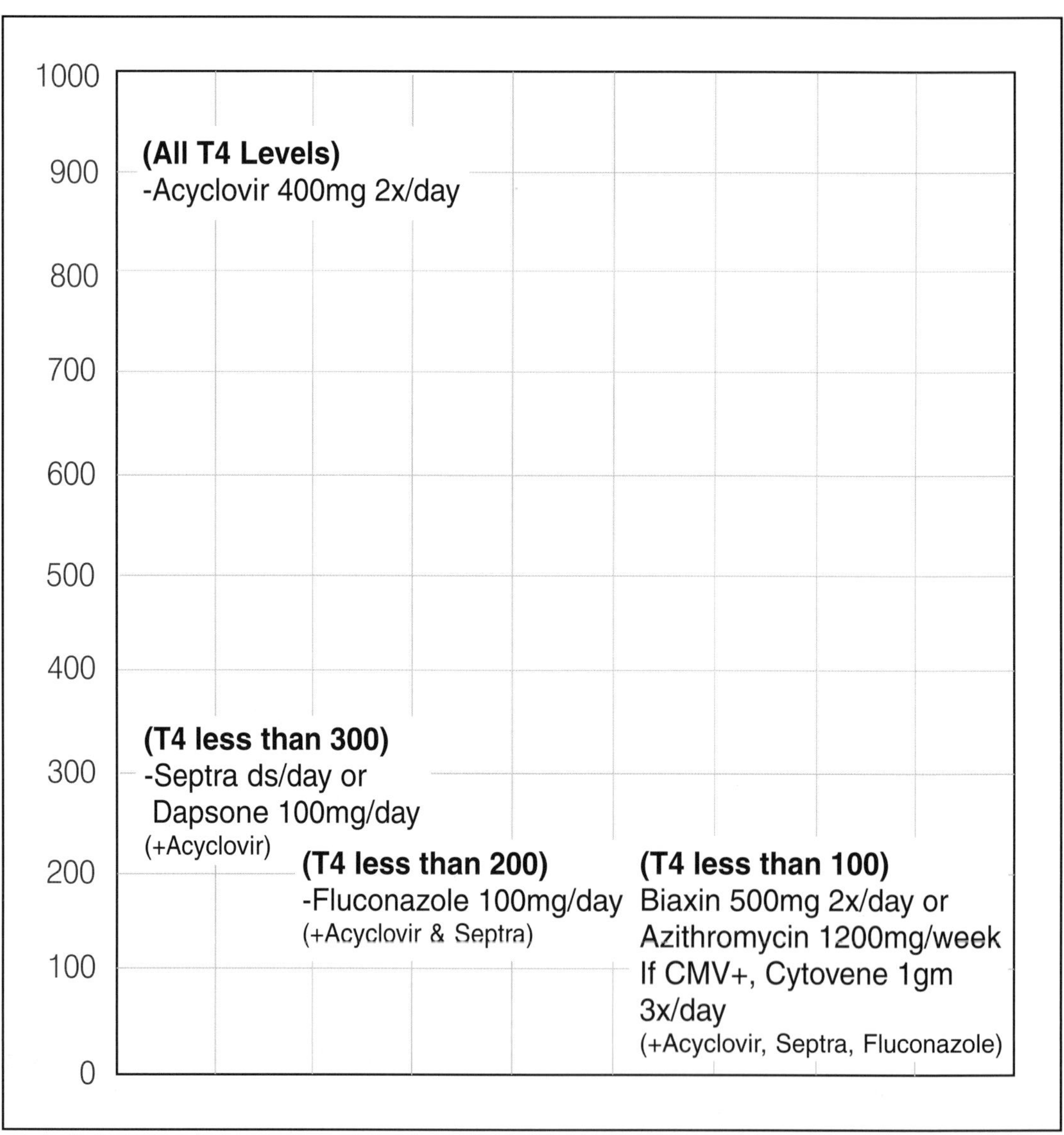

Figure 4 **The medicines to prevent the eight major Opportunistic Infections are used based on the T4 count of the patient at any given time.**

The Rule of 3 - 2- 1 guides us to provide medicines to prevent the eight major Opportunistic Infections in HIV infection as follows:

- **All people with HIV infection** should take Acyclovir at a dose of 400mg twice per day to prevent Herpes and Zoster.
- **If their T4 counts drop below 300**, then they should also take Septra ds once per day or, if they are allergic to Septra, then Dapsone at 100mg once per day to prevent PCP.
- **If their T4 counts drop below 200**, they should add Fluconazole 100mg once per day to their therapy to prevent Cryptococcus and Candida.
- Finally **if their T4 count drops below 100**, they should also take Biaxin 500mg twice per day to prevent MAI (an alternative to Biaxin is Azithromycin 1200mg taken once per week). If their urine, blood, or any other culture shows signs of CMV activity, they should add Cytovene at 1 gram three times per day to their therapy. If their blood tests show past exposure to Toxoplasma, they should be on Septra or Azithromycin.

THESE GUIDELINES ARE MORE PROTECTIVE

Readers familiar with the most common practice patterns for preventing infections in people with HIV may notice that my guidelines are more protective than other guides on HIV therapy. For instance, the most common practice is to begin medicines to prevent PCP (Pneumocystis carinii pneumonia) when the T4 count is below 200. But research in this area shows that although 95% of cases of PCP occur under a T4 count of 200, 5% occur in T4 counts between 200 and 300. My goal in more than six years of clinical practice has been to **prevent all of these potentially lethal infections** in my patients with HIV infection and not simply to follow the best cost analysis or statistical models. Therefore I suggest beginning medicines to prevent PCP if the T4 count is below 300.

Recent research has also shown another reason to be overprotective of persons with HIV and gives us strong incentive to do everything possible to prevent all Opportunistic Infections. It is now clear that HIV viral levels rise dangerously high (frequently higher than one million copies of HIV RNA/ml) if a person with HIV infection gets an Opportunistic Infection. This causes massive and rapid immune system damage and could easily lead to the rapid development of a multi-resistant HIV strain, further resulting in the collapse of the HIV therapy that the person was taking. Given this new information, sensible guidelines need to focus on preventing all of these Opportunistic Infections as the primary goal, rather than simply reducing the frequency of these infections in people with HIV.

This medication schedule listed in *Figure 3* and *Figure 4*, if properly applied, effectively prevents the eight major Opportunistic Infections (Herpes, Zoster, PCP, Cryptococcus, Candida, MAI, CMV, and Toxoplasma) in people with HIV. Less commonly, depending on where the person was born, traveled, and what infections he or she may have had, additional measures or medications may be necessary. Let's review these eight major Opportunistic Infections in detail.

HERPES

A person with HIV is at risk for recurrence of Herpes infection at all T4 levels. Herpes is a common DNA virus that forms a chronic lifelong infection in a person's facial or pelvic nerves. More than 40% of the U.S. population has had some type of Herpes infection during their lifetime. When the Herpes virus activates or "breaks out," it forms a cluster of small painful blisters on the skin. It is commonly called a "cold sore" when it occurs on the face. On the genitals it forms a similar pattern, called "genital herpes."

Herpes is typically more an annoyance than a serious infection, unless it happens to get in the eyes, where it may quickly cause permanent blindness or in the brain, where it may cause permanent brain damage or death. For people with HIV infection, Herpes can be either just a nuisance, or a major cause of facial, mouth, esophagus, genital, or perirectal ulcers. In addition, there is strong data to suggest that an active outbreak of Herpes can coactivate HIV, causing dangerously high HIV viral levels and more rapid damage to the immune system. Prevention of active Herpes infection is very important for people with HIV.

ZOSTER

At all T4 cell levels, a person with HIV is at risk of a recurrence of Chickenpox, called Zoster or Shingles. Zoster is a virus in the Herpes family. It only occurs in those people who have had Chickenpox infection during their lifetime. Zoster can come on at anytime, and happens with high frequency in people with HIV infection. It appears as a broad, deeply reddened, painful rash on one side of the body that develops from back to front following the path of the nerve it is affecting. On the rash appears hundreds of small blisters, which break to form a yellow crust, and are highly infectious to anyone who has not had Chickenpox. The pain may be moderate, but in some cases, especially if the rash breaks out on the head and face, the pain can be excruciating.

In people with HIV infection, Zoster occurs at all T4 levels, and unless prevented by medication is typically more extensive, damaging, and difficult to control and will recur relatively frequently. Like Herpes, Zoster can also coactivate HIV, dangerously increasing HIV viral levels and immune system damage during outbreaks.

PCP (Pneumocystis carinii pneumonia)

PCP occurs at T4 levels below 300, and especially below 200. In the past, this organism has been classified as a protozoa, although it has a closer genetic relationship to a fungus. By age five, most children have had PCP, which is experienced as a flu-like illness. Normally, it almost never recurs. However, if the immune system is severely weakened by HIV infection, PCP, which lies dormant in the lungs for life, may recur with a vengeance, causing rapid lung failure and death. It is also possible to be reinfected by coming in contact with another person with active PCP. National recommendations have been to start oral medicine to prevent PCP if one's T4 count is less than 200. However, the National Institutes of Health has found that although 95% of PCP cases occur below a T4 count of 200, an additional 5% occurs between a count of 200-300. I generally start prevention medicines for PCP when a T4 count drops below 300.

CRYPTOCOCCAL MENINGITIS

At T4 levels below 200, Cryptococcus neoformans may occur. Many species of birds, such as pigeons, excrete this fungus in their droppings. In time the droppings dry up, are blown around in the wind, and are inhaled by people. For a person in good health, this is not a big deal and does not cause any serious infection. However, if a person has a T4 count level that is less than 200, the inhaled fungus quickly causes a lung infection that is spread by the bloodstream to the brain lining, causing high fevers, disorientation, and severe headaches—this is called Cryptococcal meningitis. Untreated, death comes quickly. With treatment, the brain infection can be reduced, but we are not yet able to wipe out this fungal infection. An infected person will continue to have fungus in his blood and brain with mild to severe symptoms for the remainder of his life. Prevention is crucial.

CANDIDA

Candida is another fungus that is common on the skin and in the mouth of most people. It is usually only present at very low levels, but when it flares, it may cause diaper rash in babies, vaginal yeast infections in women, skin rashes in the groin area, and a mouth infection called thrush. If the immune system is normal, these are minor annoyances that resolve with minimal treatment. But if the T4 level is less than 200, the oral infection can become extensive, causing a painful infection in the mouth, throat, and esophagus. Pain can be so severe as to prevent the patient from swallowing food, or drinking.

MAI (Mycobacterium Avium Intracellulare)

Mycobacteria Avium Intracellulare/Complex (MAI/MAC) is a common bacteria found in the soil throughout the world. People with a normal immune system are rarely infected, but if their T4 count drops below 100, this bacteria can infect the lungs through inhaled dust, or the intestines through ingested soil on contaminated vegetables. In addition, if a person with HIV is working with soil, in the garden for instance, he may contaminate his hands and inadvertently ingest MAI. Once infected, MAI spreads from the lungs or gastrointestinal tract via the bloodstream to the liver, spleen, bone marrow, lymph nodes, and heart, causing fever, severe weight loss, bone marrow failure, and death. Although there is treatment for MAI infection, it is not often successful, and most people with HIV who get MAI infection die from it. The most effective way to manage MAI infection in people with HIV is to prevent them from getting it in the first place.

CMV (Cytomegalovirus)

Cytomegalovirus or CMV is a common viral infection in the general population, infecting approximately 20% to 40% of the U.S. population at sometime during their life. It is sexually transmitted like mononucleosis, and causes a flu-like illness with mild fevers, muscle aches, and fatigue lasting two to six weeks in most people. When the T4 count drops below 100, CMV may recur anywhere in the body, causing permanent blindness, pneumonia, heart failure, ulcers, paralysis, brain damage, and death.

CMV is perhaps the most lethal Opportunistic Infection for people with HIV infection and one of the most common infections in people with T4 counts below 100. Prevention is difficult—our best medicines reduce the risk of active CMV infection by only 50% at best. More effective medicines are currently under development.

TOXOPLASMA

Toxoplasma is a protozoa found in rodents, and indirectly transmitted via their droppings to grazing animals and cats. It is estimated that 20% of all pork and lamb sold in supermarkets in the U.S. is infected with Toxoplasma, but only people with weakened immune systems and pregnant women are at serious risk. If one has been infected anytime during his lifetime, Toxoplasma may recur, or if one eats undercooked or raw meat, or accidentally handles cat feces of an infected cat, primary infection may occur. With a T4 count less than 100, if a primary infection or a recurrent infection occurs, the individual commonly develops large abscesses in the brain, resulting in seizures, confusion, and, if untreated, rapid death. Toxoplasma may also occur in the lungs and in other parts of the body.

OTHER OPPORTUNISTIC INFECTIONS: TUBERCULOSIS

Tuberculosis or TB is a bacteria that can cause infection at any T4 cell level. It is a widespread infection in epidemic levels worldwide, infecting some one billion people, although it is less common in the United States. Tuberculosis forms an infection in the lungs most commonly, but may also occur in the bones, brain, abdomen, uterus, and any other part of the body. Though it is curable with triple antibiotic therapy, it can be lethal for people weakened by other illness such as HIV infection. TB is transmitted through the air, but requires prolonged exposure.

To prevent Tuberculosis, a person with HIV should avoid contact with anyone with possibly active Tuberculosis. In addition, a TB skin test should be taken every two to three years. Unfortunately the skin test is not very accurate if it is negative. As in HIV infection, the immune system may not react with a positive skin test even if the person has active Tuberculosis or has had it in the past. People with HIV infection who test positive for Tuberculosis, however, should be evaluated for active Tuberculosis by their physician.

If they have an active case of TB, they should be treated with INH, Rifampin, Pyrazinamide (or Ethambutol), and Vitamin B6 for 12 to 18 months. Always follow the most current guidelines from the Centers for Disease Control in Atlanta, Georgia as they author and frequently update the national TB treatment guidelines.

If a person with HIV has a positive TB skin test without signs of active Tuberculosis, that person should be treated with INH, Rifampin, and Vitamin B6 for a minimum of one year. Ethambutol or Pyrazinamide should be added if the person's contact for TB could possibly have been someone with resistant Tuberculosis. Again check with the Centers for Disease Control Guidelines on TB treatment.

INFECTIOUS DIARRHEA

Infectious diarrhea is common in people with HIV infection at any T4 cell level. It may be caused by many different types of organisms, including the bacteria Camplyobacter, Shigella, Salmonella, and Yersinia. These are usually acquired by ingesting contaminated food, especially undercooked or raw eggs, chicken, or shellfish, and unpasteurized dairy or juice products. These infections may also be sexually transmitted if oral/anal contamination occurs.

Amebic (Protozoal) types of infectious diarrhea include Entamoeba histolytica, Entamoeba hartmanni, Entamoeba nana, Entamoeba coli, Iodamoeba buschlii, Blastocystis, Giardia, Cryptosporidia, and Microsporidia. These are usually sexually transmitted through oral/anal contamination, but also have been transmitted through contaminated rural and city water supplies. In people with normal immune systems, they are generally not serious infections. In the setting of HIV infection, they can become chronic, and sometimes can become so serious that they cause death. Symptoms include muddy, watery, or bloody diarrhea. Infectious diarrhea caused by bacteria is most often accompanied by acute abdominal pain, fever, and blood. Amebic diarrhea (dysentery) usually causes milder symptoms, although diarrhea from Cryptosporidia or Microsporidia can be severe and even life threatening.

The best way for people with HIV infection, and all persons for that matter, to avoid infectious diarrhea is to:

- make sure all eggs, chicken, and other meat are fresh and fully cooked,
- only drink pasteurized dairy products or juices,
- make sure all water sources are purified and free of infections, and
- follow Safe Sex guidelines.

BACTERIAL PNEUMONIA

Bacterial pneumonia is fairly common in people with HIV infection, and occurs at any T4 cell level. In addition, we see more severe cases of viral pneumonia, such as Influenzae, in people with HIV. The three major bacteria that most commonly cause pneumonia in this setting are: Streptococcus pneumonia (pneumococcus), Hemophilus influenzae (a bacteria, different from Influenzae virus), and Staphlococcus aureus. Presently, there is no vaccine for Staph aureus. However there are vaccines for Strept and Hemophilus. Strept and Staph are normal bacteria in the mouth and on the skin, but in the lungs they cause serious infection. Hemophilus bacteria spreads throughout the community in the winter and spring, causing sinus, throat, ear, and lung infections in children and adults. The lung infections range from mild bronchitis to severe pneumonia. Although rare, Hemophilus may cause a brain infection called bacterial meningitis, with possible fatal outcomes. It is transmitted by hand to mouth contact.

To prevent or reduce the frequency of bacterial pneumonia and viral influenzae, people with HIV should:

- **receive Pneumococcus (Strept) vaccine at least once,** and I recommend a booster every 10 years, as people with HIV may lose immunity over time,
- **receive Hemophilus vaccine at least once.** Again I recommend a booster every 10 years,
- **receive Influenza virus vaccine every year, but not live or whole vaccine,** rather use a split or protein vaccine, and
- **do not smoke.**

CAT SCRATCH BACTERIA

A rare, but serious infection, Cat Scratch bacteria was just recently discovered and has been recently renamed Bortedella henslea. Domestic cats, and especially kittens may carry this bacteria harmlessly in their mouths or on their claws without signs of illness. If a person with HIV infection is clawed or bitten by a cat or kitten (a kitten carries a higher risk of infection), this bacteria can enter tissue and bloodstream, causing high fevers, red streaks or skin nodules, and severe illness. In its chronic phase, Cat Scratch skin nodules can look identical to the viral tumor, Kaposi's Sarcoma.

Treatment is high doses of Erythromycin for a prolonged course of treatment. **To avoid Cat Scratch infection, people with HIV should avoid scratches or bites from cats.** If you can't live without your kitty, have your veterinary doctor trim her nails every two to three weeks, or if the cat is cooperative, you can learn how to do it yourself.

HISTOPLASMA

Histoplasma, is another fungus like Cryptococcus. It is common on farms and chicken coops in the Mississippi and Ohio River Valleys, and in southern Appalachia. Many people who were brought up or lived in these rural areas experienced a flu-like illness with Histoplasma of the lungs as children. In a normally healthy person, it causes fevers, cough and a two to four week illness that resolves on its own. But if this same person becomes HIV infected and his T4 count drops below 200, or he is exposed to Histoplasma directly, infection may recur in the lungs as a lethal pneumonia, spreading to many parts of the body, including liver, spleen, blood, and bone. Unless the patient receives aggressive treatment, death is rapid.

To prevent new or recurrent Histoplasma infection, I recommend that people who live or have previously lived in endemic areas take Itraconazole 100mg once per day (instead of Fluconazole 100mg once per day) if their T4 count drops below 200.

EXAMPLE CASES

Now let's look at four individual cases and apply our 3 - 2 - 1 prevention program, first determining which Opportunistic Infections the patient is at risk for, and which medicines each should take to avoid them.

CASE 1

Subject is a 35-year-old man who grew up in New York and now lives in California. He has had no prolonged foreign travel, works now as a banker and investor, has no pets, and his T4 count one month ago was 550 cells/ml.

1. He is at risk for: **Zoster and Herpes**.

2. To prevent Zoster and Herpes, he should:
   Take Acyclovir 400mg one twice/day.

3. In addition, he should:
   - avoid contact with people with Tuberculosis and have a TB skin test every two to three years,
   - avoid undercooked food,
   - avoid smoking,
   - follow Safe Sex guidelines, and
   - vaccinate (with Pneumovax and Hemophilus vaccine every 10 years and Influenzae virus protein vaccine every year).

CASE 2

Subject is a 25-year-old woman who grew up in the Mississippi Valley. She's an aerobic instructor, currently lives in Houston. She has a healthy dog, has had no foreign travel other than to the Caribbean. Her T4 level this month is 210 cells/ml.

1. She is at risk for the following:
   - **Zoster and Herpes**, and
   - **PCP**.

2. She should do the following:
   - **Take Acyclovir** 400mg one twice/day, and
   - **Take Septra** ds one/day.

3. In addition she should:
   - avoid contact with people with Tuberculosis and have a TB skin test every two to three years,
   - avoid undercooked food,
   - avoid smoking,
   - follow Safe Sex guidelines, and
   - vaccinate (with Pneumovax and Hemophilus vaccine every 10 years and Influenzae virus protein vaccine every year).

CASE 3

Subject is 25-year-old man, who grew up in Texas and now lives in California. His only travel has been to Europe, however, his grandfather, with whom he lived for much of his childhood, recently died of Tuberculosis. All of his family has tested positive for TB, and he was treated five years ago for one year with INH/Rifampin/B6. He presently works as a computer programmer; two weeks ago his T4 count was 175. He has a healthy cat.

1. He is at risk for the following:
   - **Zoster and Herpes,**
   - **PCP,**
   - **Cryptococcal Meningitis & Candida,** and
   - **Cat Scratch Disease.**

2. He should do the following:
   - **Take Acyclovir** (400mg) one twice per day,
   - **Take Septra** ds one/day, and
   - **Take Fluconazole** (100mg) one per day.

3. In addition, he should:
   - avoid contact with people with TB,
   - avoid undercooked food,
   - avoid smoking,
   - follow Safe Sex guidelines,
   - vaccinate (with Pneumovax and Hemophilus vaccine every 10 years and Influenzae virus protein vaccine every year), and
   - avoid bites or scratches from his cat.

CASE 4

Subject is a 35-year-old man who grew up in Florida, works as a construction worker, and owns a healthy German Shepherd dog. He has traveled only to Europe and the Caribbean on short vacations, and has no known exposure to Tuberculosis. He most recent T4 count was 89 last week. He is allergic to Septra. His Toxoplasma blood test is positive, but he has no signs of active Toxoplasma infection.

1. He is at risk for:
   - **Zoster and Herpes,**
   - **PCP,**
   - **Cryptococcal Meningitis & Candida,**
   - **MAI,**
   - **CMV,** and
   - **recurrent Toxoplasma Infection.**

2. He should do the following:
   - **Acyclovir** (400mg) one twice per day,
   - **Dapsone** (100mg) one per day (he is allergic to Septra),
   - **Fluconazole** (100mg) one per day,
   - **Azithromycin** (250mg) one twice per day (chosen to simultaneously prevent MAI and Toxo), and
   - have a blood or urine test for CMV done every three months (his last two months ago was negative).

3. In addition, he should:
   - avoid contact with people with Tuberculosis and have a TB skin test every two to three years,
   - avoid undercooked food,
   - avoid direct contact with soil,

- avoid smoking,
- follow Safe Sex guidelines, and
- vaccinate (with Pneumovax and Hemophilus vaccine every 10 years and Influenzae virus protein vaccine every year.

WHAT TO DO WHEN A LOW T4 COUNT INCREASES SUBSTANTIALLY?

First of all, celebrate! There is too much pessimism in the field. People with low T4 counts who go into Remission through effective triple therapy (as confirmed by a consistently zero or undetectable HIV levels) have dramatic and sustained improvements in their health. Many serious infections such as CMV, MAI, and even very rare but lethal infections such as PML of the brain frequently resolve. The health changes that we see when a person with HIV is placed in Remission on triple therapy are among the most astounding recoveries from severe illness ever reported in modern medicine.

THE "BAD" T4 CELL RUMOR

There are rumors that strong T4 counts that have risen as a result of triple therapy don't have as much effect as the same T4 counts in people taking no HIV treatment. The opposite is true. A person on no therapy with a T4 count of, say 450, and an HIV level of 100,000 likely has a **weaker** immune system than a person on triple therapy whose T4 count has risen to 450 with an HIV level of zero. In the person on no treatment, the majority of T4 cells are likely in the process of being HIV-infected and therefore becoming nonfunctional. In the person with a T4 count of 450 and an HIV level of zero, all the available T4 cells are uninfected and remain completely functional. The reports of recurrent Opportunistic Infections at high T4 cells in people recovering from HIV are exceedingly rare, and are being overwhelmed by reports of astounding, sustained improvements in health, and concurrent resolution of previously lethal Opportunistic Infections as a result of effective treatment. These rare reports of Opportunistic Infections at higher than expected T4 counts more likely represent closer observations of rare, but well known deviations from average patterns ("the bell curve") that occurs in all diseases.

DELETING PREVENTION MEDICINES

May we delete medicines as the T4 count rises? This is an area of controversy. Over my years of experience treating people with HIV with combination therapy and more than one year since the advent of triple therapy, I have deleted prevention medicines as my patient's T4 counts have risen. If a person's T4 count of 50 rises and remains above 100, the prevention for MAI and CMV may stopped. As T4 counts rise above 200, Fluconazole (prevention for Cryptococcus and Candida) may be deleted, and as counts rise above 300, Septra (prevention for PCP) may be deleted. My patients have remained healthy and I have seen no unusual patterns of Opportunistic Infections in more than six years of experience. But this area of treatment is new and deserves vigilant study.

THE RULE OF 3 - 2 - 1 ONLY APPLIES TO PREVENTION

If a person has active CMV, active MAI, active Cryptococcus, or another active infection, the situation is very different. The changes in therapy in these cases are not clear. **I am not addressing treatment of active Opportunistic Infections in this book,** although that may be an interesting subject for another book.

In my practice, I generally treat active infections until every test and scan are negative, and every symptom and sign of the infection has returned to normal. Then and only then will I consider backing off on the treatment of active infections, and even then I proceed with caution. Thus, a person with a T4 count of 50 who gets active CMV of the retina, and whose T4 count rises to 200 in the course of treatment for CMV would continue that treatment for an uncertain period of time based on the case, the location of the infection, the type of infection, and follow-up exams and tests to determine the status of the infection.

However, a person who has never had an active infection with CMV, whose T4 count was 50, and now rises to 200, who is on effective triple therapy with a zero HIV level, could stop CMV prevention, MAI prevention, and Cyptococcus and Candida prevention. Based on the rule of 3 - 2 - 1, **a person who has never had any of these infections** would only need to take prevention for PCP, Herpes, and Zoster. Besides their triple therapy, they would need only Septra ds once per day and Acyclovir 400mg twice per day.

SUMMARY

We have reached an era in which more than 90% of Opportunistic Infections in people with HIV can be avoided or prevented. The basic techniques to preventing infections are to:

- take specific medicines to prevent the eight Opportunistic Infections based on the T4 count at a given time, according to the rule of 3 - 2 - 1,
- avoid of sources of infections,
- avoid of raw or undercooked foods,
- avoid scratches or bites from cats or kittens,
- avoid soil contact (if the T4 count is less than 100).

The Rule of 3 - 2 - 1 is a simple, broad guideline that effectively prevents Opportunistic Infections in people with HIV. With it a person with HIV can easily form a sensible treatment plan with his or her doctor that prevents almost all major infections.

8
REVERSING WASTING SYNDROME

8 REVERSING WASTING SYNDROME

"SLIM DISEASE"

Another of the three focal points in the treatment of HIV infection is the treatment of Wasting Syndrome, defined as an involuntary loss of 10% or more of lean body weight with weakness, diarrhea, or fever. This condition is common worldwide in people with HIV infection. In Africa, it's called "Slim Disease." Past studies have shown that fully 63% of people with HIV have some level of malnutrition, and 21% have Wasting Syndrome.

People with severe Wasting Syndrome resemble starvation victims with gaunt, drawn faces, thin limbs, and skeletal torsos, devoid of muscle. But the condition is not simply cosmetic—it is one of the most serious and lethal conditions associated with HIV infection. Untreated, people with Wasting Syndrome exceed a 50% death rate per year, and have a mean life span of 14 months. People with Wasting Syndrome suffer excessively and the syndrome affects all major systems of the body.

SYMPTOMS

Typical symptoms of Wasting Syndrome, besides excessive weight loss include:

- severe fatigue,
- nausea,
- confusion and disorientation,
- frequent infections that respond poorly to therapy,
- depression,
- altered bowel patterns, either diarrhea or constipation,
- muscle aches and diffuse pain syndromes.

WASTING DRAINS THE IMMUNE SYSTEM

The malnutrition that accompanies Wasting Syndrome causes the immune system, already severely impaired by HIV, to function at an even lower level, and it causes a reduction in cellular replication rate, which means one's T4 count drops more rapidly than it would otherwise. In addition, the immune system cells that are produced fail to respond quickly to fight infections. Healing is severely impaired, and the body does not clear infections at a normal rate, despite appropriate antibiotics. Other factors being equal, people with Wasting Syndrome have more frequent infections, respond poorly to treatment, and have a higher death rate per year than people with HIV infection who are not wasted.

WASTING SYNDROME IS TREATABLE

Most physicians and health care workers who treat people with HIV infection consider Wasting Syndrome, or weight loss, untreatable and an inevitable part of HIV disease. Typically, little effort is made to identify, stop, or reverse this condition, and there are currently no standardized plans to treat it. Today an estimated 200,000 people suffer with Wasting Syndrome in the United States alone, and with it they suffer from its associated impairments, decreased quality of life, social stigma, and high death rate.

It is not sufficient to ask a person if he or she is eating. I find it most useful to ask **what** the person ate in the last 24 hours, make a quick list, and estimate the total calories per day.

CALORIE REQUIREMENTS ARE HIGH

To maintain weight a person with HIV needs a minimum of 2000 calories per day, which is three large meals with snacks. **To gain weight**, if no other problems exist (infection, tumor, diarrhea), that person must eat almost 3000 calories per day. There are many misconceptions about HIV and Wasting Syndrome. The facts are:

- Wasting Syndrome is **not** an inevitable part of HIV and AIDS.
- Wasting Syndrome is **not** untreatable.
- Weight is **not** permanently lost in this condition. Muscle cell numbers generally remain unchanged, although the muscle cell volume decreases, which causes generalized body muscle atrophy.
- AZT does **not** cause Wasting Syndrome, as previously thought. There is a very rare condition of AZT-induced muscle inflammation (myositis),

which is easily diagnosed based on diffuse muscle tenderness and elevated blood CPK. This condition reverses within one to two weeks of stopping AZT, and occurs in less than 5% of those people who use AZT.

- Simply eating more food does **not** usually solve Wasting Syndrome.
- HIV does **not** typically cause fevers. With the exception of a brief period of fevers during the initial infection with HIV, almost all fevers in HIV are caused by a new or recurrent infection, tumor, or drug allergy.
- HIV does **not** typically cause diarrhea. Diarrhea in HIV is almost always due to undiagnosed infection, many very difficult to identify.

IDENTIFYING WASTING SYNDROME

All people with HIV infection should be monitored every three to six months for weight loss and Wasting Syndrome. Like any condition in medicine, the sooner a problem is identified, the easier it is to treat and reverse the problem.

The goal is to maintain appropriate ideal body weight. Since most people with HIV infection malabsorb fat, they generally have lower blood cholesterol levels and are generally not obese. Their measured scale weights are considered to approximate lean body weight.

IDEAL BODY WEIGHT

The individual's scale weight and height are measured. In addition, ask for and note the minimum and maximum weights over the past five years. Next, determine the individual's **Ideal Body Weight**, using standard medical calculations [*see Figure 1*].

CALCULATING IDEAL BODY WEIGHT (IBW)

1. Record the person's height.
2. Count the number of inches above five feet.
3. **For men, IBW = 106 pounds + (6 x inches above 5 feet)**.
4. **For women, IBW = 104 pounds + (4 x inches above 5 feet).**
5. Adjust by plus or minus 10% based on whether the individual is large framed, average framed, or slender framed.

Figure 1 **The Ideal Body Weight (IBW) is calculated by determining the individual's height and weight and using the above equations.**

Let's examine two cases and determine Ideal Body Weight and the extent of Wasting Syndrome.

CASE 1

A large-framed man who is 6' 1" is analyzed to determine Ideal Body Weight. His current weight is 145 lb. His maximum weight over the past five years was 220 lb. and his minimum weight is his current weight of 145 lb.. At 6' 1", he is 13 inches taller than five feet. Therefore, the calculated **Ideal Body Weight** for this person is 106 lb. + (6 x 13) = 106 + 78 = 184 lb. However, since this man is large framed, 10% more is added to the calculated weight or 184 + 18.4 = 202.4 lb. This person has Wasting Syndrome and is 202 lb. minus 145 lb. = 57 lb. lower than his Ideal Body Weight.

CASE 2

Here's a second example: An average framed 30-year-old woman with HIV infection who is 5' 6" is analyzed to determine Ideal Body Weight. Her current weight is 98 lb. Her maximum weight over the past five years was 160 lb. and her minimum weight was 85 lb. At 5' 6", she is six inches above five feet in height. Therefore, her calculated **Ideal Body Weight** is 104 lb. + (4 x 6) = 104 + 24 = 128 lb. Since she is of average frame, no adjustment is made. She has Wasting Syndrome and is 128 lb. minus 98 lb. = 30 lb. below her Ideal Body Weight.

THREE CAUSES OF WASTING

There are three basic causes of Wasting Syndrome (weight loss) in people with HIV infection:

- an unidentified medical problem,
- lack of sufficient calorie (food) intake, and
- hormone deficiency.

AN UNIDENTIFIED MEDICAL PROBLEM

An unidentified medical problem, which can be infection, tumor, or infectious or non-infectious diarrhea, manifests itself as Wasting Syndrome because large amounts of calories or nutrition are diverted to fight the problem rather than going toward body maintenance.

INFECTION

To fight an infection, the body diverts large amounts of calories or nutrition to mobilize the immune system. In addition, metabolic rate is greatly increased on a cellular level, as well as in mounting a fever, fast heart rate, fast breathing rate, more rapid functioning of liver and kidney systems, and increased glandular function (especially of the thyroid and adrenal systems).

TUMOR

Tumors or cancer in HIV is a group of conditions where normal human cells become altered to grow at high rates without respect to tissue boundaries. These cells have high calorie needs due to their high growth rate, and literally use up calories from the blood that supplies them. Common tumors or cancers in HIV infection are lymphoma, leukemia, rectal cancer, and Kaposi's Sarcoma (KS). Interestingly, KS is considered a viral sarcoma because it is caused by a virus, Herpes type 8, but grows like a tumor.

DIARRHEA

Diarrhea prevents calories or nutrition from being absorbed into the body and causes the most calorie loss in HIV. Diarrhea in HIV is usually caused by an infection of the gastrointestinal tract, such as bacteria (Salmonella, Shigella, Yersinia, Campylobacter), protozoa (Giardia, Entamoeba species, Cryptosporidia, Microsporidia), virus (CMV, Adenovirus, Norwalk virus, Rotavirus), or tumor (intestinal KS, lymphoma), and less rarely, fungi.

FINDING THE ANSWER

A person with HIV who begins to have abrupt and rapid weight loss, frequently a loss of 10 or more pounds within a two to four week period, almost always has a new or recurrent infection, tumor, or diarrhea syndrome. Common infections that are difficult to identify in their early stages include PCP, CMV of any site, Tuberculosis, Cat Scratch Disease, MAI, Toxoplasmosis, and fungal infections such as Aspergillis and Mucor. Common tumors are lymphoma, leukemia, and KS. The more elusive diarrhea syndromes to identify are Giardia, Cryptosporidia, Microsporidia, and CMV or MAI enteritis.

Symptoms, besides abrupt and rapid weight loss, may include new fatigue, fevers, night sweats, headaches, cough, nausea, vomiting, pain, skin changes, uncontrollable diarrhea, and enlarging lymph nodes, liver, or spleen.

If a standard exam and blood tests do not reveal the source of infection, some tests that are helpful are serum LDH, sedimentation rate, serum Toxoplasma IgG/ IgM, serum Cryptococcal antigen, blood cultures for bacteria, virus, fungus, and AFB, stool for Giardia, ova and parasite, C. difficile toxin, Cryptosporidia, Microsporidia, bacterial, viral, AFB, and fungal stains and cultures. Of course, not all of these tests need to be done. Select based on the details of the particular case.

If these results do not reveal the source, either do a full body Gallium scan or a CT or MRI of any area of pain or problems. Plan to biopsy any abscess, mass, or highlighted, inflamed areas that show up on these imaging studies. If diarrhea is the primary symptom and stool cultures are unrevealing, proceed with a colonoscopy with biopsies and cultures to obtain the cause of the diarrhea. The goal is to find the answer within one to two weeks and treat as soon as possible.

LACK OF SUFFICIENT CALORIE INTAKE

The second cause of Wasting Syndrome in HIV is lack of sufficient calorie intake, a very obvious cause of weight loss that is frequently overlooked in HIV. Some cases involve people who are **unable to eat** due to oral ulcers or teeth pain. Others are **unable to swallow** due to ulcers or infections of the esophagus. Some are **unable retain food in their stomach** due to nausea, vomiting, or stomach pain, which itself may be attributable to a variety of causes, including ulcers, tumors, infections, and medications.

But these are relatively easy to evaluate and treat. An endoscopy, where a Gastroenterologist briefly places a small scope into the esophagus and stomach, is often useful for quickly identifying the problem.

However, it's not uncommon for people with HIV infection to have a normal endoscopy and still complain of nausea or lack of appetite. Medications, in particular HIV medicines such as AZT and Ritonavir, and many antimicrobials such as Flagyl, Humatin, Foscarnet, and Amphotericin may cause nausea. You must identify the medicine causing the problem and find an alternative. Simple nausea may be treated with medicines such as Compazine, Ativan, Zofran, Kytril, Marinol, and marijuana derivatives (marijuana derivatives should only be used if available and not legally problematic). In addition, for those with Wasting Syndrome and appropriate medical needs, replacement testosterone and its derivative, Nandrolone, enhance appetite greatly.

DEPRESSION MAY CAUSE WEIGHT LOSS

Depression may also be a cause of insufficient calorie intake. Depression is common in severe disease, especially HIV. The causes of depression are usually very basic and include major problems in one or more of five areas: health, social (loss/isolation), living situation, financial difficulties, or employment.

Undergoing a brief period of supportive therapy can be very helpful. Antidepressant medications such as Prozac, Paxil, Wellbutrin, Serzone, Trazadone, and Nortriptyline are among a few that may help during severe depression, elevating one's mood enough so that one can think clearly, reorganize issues, and then possibly begin to solve them through the assistance of therapy, friends, a physician, and/or social organizations. Medications provide prompt benefit—within one to two weeks. The process of solving depression with intensive therapy and organization may take six months or more.

Social isolation is common among people with HIV infection and can directly cause depression. Men and women with HIV should be encouraged to participate in social activities such as sports, and other social events, and they should be encouraged to gain and maintain close friendships and relationships.

INABILITY TO OBTAIN FOOD

Obviously, for people without financial means to obtain food, lack of money is an obvious cause of weight loss and Wasting Syndrome, but there are frequently more subtle causes. People with severe HIV infection (AIDS) are often fatigued and may have difficulty walking to the food store, or standing to prepare food. Ask to determine if this is the case and refer this person to a social service that can help.

HORMONE DEFICIENCY

The third major cause of Wasting Syndrome is hormone deficiency, a relatively new and helpful discovery in the field of HIV. It occurs more often in men than women, 10% of the time when the T4 count is greater than 300 cells/ml and about 30% of the time when the T4 count is less than 300. Although this information has been well published in the scientific literature—it was first described approximately five years ago—most physicians and health care workers have very little knowledge or experience in identifying hormone deficiency, or treating it.

The deficiency occurs in the form of hypogonadism or gonadal failure. The reasons for this deficiency are not yet clear, although it is well established that the gonads are very sensitive to acute and chronic infections, especially viral infections. In addition, HIV is primarily and heavily found in semen which originates from the male gonads and prostate glands. Medicines that are used to treat primary HIV infection may also suppress gonadal function, although the condition has been described in people on therapy, as well as in people who have elected no therapy. We are just beginning to understand that the gonads are much more than organs of sexual reproduction. The testes in men and the ovaries in women provide hormones, or chemical signals, that are sent into the blood stream on a continuous basis affecting the function of many bodily systems.

TESTOSTERONE

The primary hormone in men is testosterone. Its many benefits include sexual function, sexual libido, maintenance of lean body weight, maintenance of a strong and rapid immune system response, and assistance in maintaining a normal mood.

ESTROGEN

Similarly, in women, the primary hormone estrogen provides many benefits including sexual function, sexual libido (although endogenous female testosterone may play a stronger role), maintenance of body weight, maintenance of a strong immune system response, and maintenance of a normal mood.

THE DIAGNOSIS OF HYPOGONADISM

The diagnosis of hypogonadism in people with HIV infection is relatively straight forward. In males, look for persistent loss of libido, persistent loss of sexual function, primary muscle atrophy, malaise, depression, and lassitude.

In females the symptoms may be more subtle: changes in libido, primary muscle atrophy, loss of overlying skin fat layer (despite sufficient food intake), irregular (or no) menstrual cycles, dry skin, and thinning hair.

Work up consists of a patient interview followed by appropriate hormone blood tests. In men, hypogonadism is established by a serum total testosterone level less than 300mg/dl (varies by lab), regardless of symptoms. Some groups also look at serum testosterone percent and free testosterone. Suspect hypogonadism if the serum total testosterone is less than 400mg/dl and all symptoms are present. Replacement hormone treatment should be initiated within one month of diagnosis and is required lifelong. For women, consult a Gynecologist. Blood tests for serum estrogen, progestin, FSH, and LH may be done on day one, day 15, and day 30 if necessary to establish the diagnosis.

TREATMENT FOR HYPOGONADISM

For men, treatment is **testosterone enanthate: 300 to 500mg by intramuscular injection every two weeks, or testosterone patches: two-2.5mg patches applied every day to the skin.**

For women, **treatment is estrogen/progestin as prescribed by a gynecologist.** Use of low dose testosterone is not recommended in women due to multiple side effects, including growth of facial hair and deepening of voice.

Hypogonadism or gonadal hormone deficiency is especially common among males with HIV infection due to impairment or damage to the testes resulting in an abnormally low testosterone level. In my practice, I have found it to be **the major cause of chronic weight loss**. But replacement is easy and works in virtually every case. Replacement is also very low cost. The cost of injectable testosterone rarely exceeds $40 per month. Estrogen/progestin replacement is also generic and even less costly.

Since replacement brings a person's low hormone levels to previously normal levels, there are virtually no side effects, although occasionally with injectable testosterone, there is slight, transient tenderness at the injection site for one to two days after the injection, and people using the testosterone skin patches may have a minor skin reaction. If dosed too high, testosterone can cause acne, alopecia (balding), and rarely, breast development or nodules. Thus treatment should follow recommended guidelines.

With appropriate replacement, sexual function returns to normal, weight increases, and mood normalizes. Most people with Wasting Syndrome due to hypogonadism regain all their lost weight within one to two months. It is not uncommon to gain anywhere from five to 20 pounds of lean body weight without much effort.

Other therapies have been proposed by various research groups for Wasting Syndrome but I believe that many of them are not useful, and some appear prone to side effects, or to an unfortunate pharmaceutical effort to financially exploit people with HIV. Some of these proposed therapies include Megase, Growth Hormone, and Thalidomide.

MEGASE

Megase, or Megesterol acetate is a prescription medicine similar to corticosteroid and used in breast cancer. Research on people with HIV initially demonstrates mild gains in appetite and weight. However, further research published in the Annals of Internal Medicine shows that this weight is mainly salt and water, and that the drug frequently suppresses a key gland of the body, the adrenal gland.

Megase is not useful for the treatment of HIV Wasting Syndrome and may even be harmful. People with HIV should not use Megase and the FDA should rescind its approval of the use of Megase for HIV Wasting.

GROWTH HORMONE

Human Growth Hormone, hGH, is a genetically cloned hormone approved for treatment of people with HIV and Wasting Syndrome. Weight gain on daily injections of growth hormone was dismal in clinical trials, averaging 3.5 lb. over a three month period at a pharmacy cost of $12,000.

And growth hormone is not present in adults at any significant level. If growth hormone is accidentally produced by a tumor, it produces a potentially lethal condition, called Acromegaly. Acromegaly causes excessive bone and cartilage growth in the forehead, nose, ears, and hands. "Lurch" in the Adams Family show and "Jaws" in the James Bond movie had the characteristics of Acromegaly. It also causes diabetes and heart enlargement. Untreated, people with Acromegaly die an early death.

In addition, although it is not much different in structure than insulin (which costs pennies to make), the company making growth hormone charges more than $4000 per month and more than $50,000 per year for the drug. Given its poor performance in clinical trials, the potential risk of serious long term side effects, and its excessively high cost, there are better alternatives for the treatment of Wasting Syndrome than growth hormone.

THALIDOMIDE

Thalidomide is an older drug that was withdrawn from the market due to severe birth defects. Recently there has been some interest in its use for Wasting Syndrome. It is unclear what mechanism of action it would play in reversing Wasting Syndrome, and initial results have been marginal at best. As it has caused serious birth defects in the past, it may be capable of causing genetic damage in adults, which could result in higher incidence of cancer, especially lymphoma and leukemia. I view Thalidomide with much caution, and believe it has very little potential benefit.

NEW THERAPIES FOR WASTING

There are two new therapies that are very helpful in increasing lean body weight in men with HIV infection who are eating well, have no other underlying condition, and do not regain all of their weight if testosterone replacement is appropriate and initiated. They are Nandrolone and Oxandrolone.

NANDROLONE

Nandrolone is a synthetic derivative of testosterone. It provides all testosterone's benefits with an enhanced effect in gains in lean body weight. It is generic and costs approximately $40 per month. Weight gain is immediate, and enhanced if the person exercises and eats 2000 to 3000 calories per day. Nandrolone is in the same base mix as testosterone enanthate and may be mixed in the same syringe. A common therapy might be either:

Nandrolone 200 to 300mg by injection every two weeks, or

testosterone 300mg-400mg + Nandrolone 200mg every two weeks.

until the desired weight is gained. At that point the therapy may be stopped or reduced to testosterone replacement only, if the person has an underlying testosterone deficiency. Side effects are rare. Like testosterone, if Nandrolone is used at too high a dose, facial, back, and chest acne may occur. Temporary impotence may occur if Nandrolone is used without supplemental testosterone for more than two months. At high doses, side effects such as acne, alopecia, breast development or nodules, or even harmful enlargement of the heart muscle could occur.

Although generic and FDA approved, research of Nandrolone in HIV Wasting is ongoing. Some of the best clinicians treating people with HIV have been using this therapy for more than three years with great success and no significant side effects to my knowledge. However, dosing should not exceed amounts listed and should be used only when appropriate. Nandrolone therapy should not exceed more than six months during a year of therapy, until further research is completed on the long term effects of continuous Nandrolone therapy.

OXANDROLONE

Oxandrolone (Oxandrin) is basically Nandrolone in pill form. Dosing is two 5mg pills twice or three times per day. Oxandrin should have the same benefits as Nandrolone, and the minimal research that has been done suggests good gains in lean body weight. Side effects risks are similar to those of testosterone and Nandrolone. At approved doses, the medicine appears safe and effective. Used alone without supplemental testosterone temporary impotence may occur by month two or three. However, although the medication costs pennies to make, and the manufacturer has minimal investment in drug development and research, it is charging approximately $700 per month for a standard dose. With an equivalent medicine Nandrolone costing $40 per month it is difficult to recommend Oxandrin, when the excess funds would be better spent on a Protease Inhibitor or other necessary treatment.

SUMMARY

Wasting Syndrome is serious and sometimes lethal but it is treatable and should be reversible in **all** cases. Its three causes are:

- **unidentified medical problem,**
- **lack of sufficient calorie (food) intake, and**
- **hormone deficiency (hypogonadism).**

Testosterone deficiency is common in men with HIV. **Treatment is replacement testosterone 300 to 500mg by intramuscular injection every two weeks.**

Ovarian failure may also occur in women with HIV but is less common. **Treatment is replacement estrogen/progestin.**

If additional weight gain is desirable for men with Wasting, new therapies include:

- **Nandrolone 200 to 300mg by injection every two weeks,**
- **testosterone 300mg-400mg + Nandrolone 200mg every two weeks,**
- **Oxandrolone two 5mg pills twice per day.**

9
ECONOMICS OF HIV HEALTH CARE

9 ECONOMICS OF HIV HEALTH CARE

EPIDEMICS ARE EMERGENCIES

The price tag for treatment of HIV infection has been a focus of discussion in almost every research conference or clinical meeting to date. Indeed, in many regions of the United States, cost is the driving factor for when, how, and to what extent people with HIV are treated. In other epidemics such as Polio or Tuberculosis, cost discussions were integral to public policy planning, but did not to any extent influence the recommendations for treatment strategy. In these cases, budget requests made of the government were simply for delivering the most effective therapy to the public at large.

IT'S MORE COSTLY TO WAIT

Unfortunately, current economic discussions on local and national treatment models for HIV/AIDS are heavily influenced by a policy of neglect and bigotry towards the groups that HIV/AIDS most heavily affects. The consensus is that it is too expensive to treat HIV/AIDS. I propose, as do many in the field currently, that the contrary is true: it's too costly not to properly treat persons with HIV/AIDS. The price of our current policies of neglect are many, including the enormous price of disability and terminal illness, the price of a spreading, ever increasing epidemic, the price to the economy and the country of lost talent and lives, and the immeasurable price of human pain and suffering.

THREE MODELS FOR HIV/AIDS

Let's consider the economics of HIV/AIDS by looking at three treatment models characterized by:

- delayed treatment,
- mid disease non-aggressive treatment, or
- early, aggressive treatment.

MODEL 1, DELAYED TREATMENT

Delayed treatment has been the primary model in place over the 15 years of the epidemic and is only recently being replaced by Model 2. Delayed treatment consists of a "wait and see" approach, and incredibly, is still advocated by some national leaders. In this model, people with HIV take no or very minimal medications, and only receive treatment for serious infections, or when they become ill.

It has been well established that more than 95% of people with HIV infection will become seriously ill and die within two to 15 years of their initial infection if they don't receive effective triple therapy. Anyone following this model will predictably have multiple life threatening infections and cancers, and will eventually enter a terminal phase of medical care. The terminal phase lasts an average of one to two years in this model. Then the person dies.

THE COSTS OF MODEL 1

The costs are among the highest in all of medical care. Hospitalizations typically cost $20,000 to $50,000 each. If terminal care involves an Intensive Care Unit, the tab may tip $100,000 per admission. *Figure 1* represents a cost analysis based on an average course of illness of a person who elects this treatment approach.

MODEL 2, MID DISEASE, NON-AGGRESSIVE TREATMENT

Mid disease, non-aggressive treatment is the predominant model in use in the U. S. today. Model 2 proposes to begin treatment when the T4 count drops below 500. A non-aggressive approach is taken, which means single or combination antiviral therapy. This therapy is only marginally and temporarily beneficial. After short periods of time HIV breaks through the therapy, and after two to four years typically forms a multi-resistant strain, which does not respond to any HIV therapy.

THE COSTS OF HIV/AIDS BASED ON MODEL 1, DELAYED TREATMENT

1. Two episodes of Pneumocyctis carinii pneumonia, both requiring hospitalization.	**$40,000**
2. Chronic Esophageal Candida, which becomes resistant, requiring Amphotericen therapy.	**$50,000**
3. Multiple episodes of CMV retinitis, resulting in partial blindness.	**$100,000**
4. Cryptococcal meningitis and pneumonia	**$30,000**
5. Terminal phase Wasting and Pneumocystis carinii pneumonia with Intensive Care Unit, intubation (respirator), bilateral pneumothoracies, sepsis, and death.	**$100,000**
6. Miscellaneous outpatient medications, doctor visits home nursing, home attendant care, and Emergency room visits.	**$50,000**
The estimated total expenses for this approach is:	**$370,000**

Figure 1 **The costs of patient care for Model 1, Delayed Treatment are very high due to recurrent severe illness, hospitalization, and terminal care. In addition, during the final two year phase of this person's life, he or she went through incalculable pain, debilitation, and suffering, which is not measurable by costing data.**

MODEL 2 ENCOURAGES MULTI-RESISTANT HIV

As the multi-resistant HIV strains emerge, the immune system (as measured by the T4 count) begins to fail. As the T4 count drops below 200, the infected person begins to have multiple Opportunistic Infections, and will require many medications in an attempt to prevent other infections from occurring. This situation worsens as the T4 count drops below 100.

Most commonly, the final phase in these cases involves the two most deadly infections associated with HIV/AIDS, which are CMV (Cytomegalovirus) and MAI (Mycobacterium Avium Intracellulare). Either causes suffering and debilitation. One goes through a protracted period of hospitalizations, and requires intravenous and oral medications. Death usually occurs with partial or full blindness due to CMV, severe wasting due to MAI, CMV, or Cryptosporidiosis, and in 10% to 40% of cases brain disease caused by CMV, HIV, Cryptococcus, PML, Toxoplasmosis, or lymphoma.

THE COSTS OF MODEL 2

The costs are the highest of all the models because Model 2's soft approach allows HIV to become slowly but progressively multi-resistant. A non-aggressive approach produces responses to therapy that are initially encouraging, with good T4 responses and low HIV levels. However, after a short period of time HIV breaks through each therapy and no longer responds to any medicines. This model also includes a terminal disease phase as in Model 1. Its members ultimately fail therapy, become progressively ill, and then die of HIV/AIDS. The costs are itemized in *Figure 2*.

MODEL 3, EARLY AGGRESSIVE TREATMENT

Model 3 is the model that leading scientists and clinicians in the field have been proposing and using. It consists of aggressive and early treatment for all people with HIV infection regardless of their T4 count or HIV level. Dr. David Ho of the Aaron Diamond Research Institute in New York put succinctly:

"Treat Early, Treat Hard"

The goal of Model 3 is to completely "shut off" HIV infection and place HIV in Remission. If HIV is not actively replicating, it cannot become resistant, and the emergence of multi-resistant HIV strains is halted. One does not progress to AIDS. Indeed, in my years of experience with this type of treatment, almost everyone's health returns to normal and they lead essentially normal and productive lives.

THE COSTS OF HIV/AIDS BASED ON MODEL 2, MID PHASE, NON-AGGRESSIVE THERAPY

1. Six years of non-aggressive single or combination therapy at $5000 per year per person.	**$30,000**
2. Two episodes of Pneumocyctis carinii pneumonia, both requiring hospitalization.	**$40,000**
3. Chronic Esophageal Candidiasis which becomes resistant, requiring Amphotericen therapy.	**$50,000**
4. Multiple episodes of CMV retinitis, resulting in partial blindness.	**$100,000**
5. Cryptococcal meningitis and pneumonia	**$30,000**
6. Terminal phase Wasting and Pneumocystis carinii pneumonia with Intensive Care Unit, intubation (respirator), bilateral pneumothoracies, sepsis and death.	**$100,000**
7. Miscellaneous outpatient medications, doctor visits home nursing, home attendant care, and Emergency room visits.	**$50,000**
The estimated total expenses for this approach is:	**$400,000**

Figure 2 **The costs of Model 2 are the highest of all HIV/AIDS treatment models due to the emergence of multi-resistant HIV infection, multiple hospitalizations and terminal care.**

THE COSTS OF MODEL 3

The costs for this model are surprisingly low. Therapy involves triple therapy--three simultaneous HIV medicines administered together to fully stop HIV replication. Current costs for most Nucleoside Analog medications (AZT, d4T, ddI, 3TC, ddC) are approximately $200 per month (based on rates negotiated by most medical insurance). The costs of the most effective and safe Protease Inhibitors, Nelfinavir and Crixivan, are $460 and $390 per month respectively.

New medicines should not exceed $400 to $500 per month for those with complex manufacturing processes, and $200 per month for those that are relatively simple to manufacture. With a wider audience, volume discounts would be sensible, and the pharmaceutical industry could recoup their research expenses through volume sales at low costs rather than limited sales at high prices.

In this model, the total costs are approximately that of the medicines as hospitalizations virtually disappear, and in general patients on this therapy have no more serious complications than the general public. People with HIV who receive early aggressive therapy need only see their physicians four to six times per year, making doctors costs minimal. These costs are itemized in *Figure 3*.

THE COSTS OF HIV/AIDS BASED ON MODEL 3, EARLY AGGRESSIVE TREATMENT

1. Ten years of aggressive triple therapy at $900/month	**$108,000**
2. Ten years of doctor office visits four to six times per year at $80 per visit.	**$4800**
The estimated total expenses for this approach is:	**$112,800**

Figure 3 **The costs of Model 3 are approximately the costs of HIV medicines, as hospitalizations and complications are virtually nonexistent.**

Model 3 is clearly the most cost effective treatment plan, saving 60% to 80% over the others. And I have an idea for what to do with the money saved. Put it toward a Manhattan style "cure project," to find a treatment to rid people of the HIV virus entirely, which would allow them to completely stop therapy. Given our current knowledge of HIV, and the current state of technology, it is likely that a fully funded project involving America's best scientists could produce a cure for those infected and a vaccine against further spread of HIV within five years, which would ultimately mean the end of the most deadly world epidemic of our era.

A NATIONAL HIV/AIDS TREATMENT PROGRAM

Epidemics have characteristics that can only be successfully addressed on a national and international level due to their broad scope and population dynamics. Like wars, epidemics are a public policy issue. There are many precedents for a National Treatment Program for HIV/AIDS. Polio and Tuberculosis come to mind most readily. Other epidemics and public health issues where national programs have been instituted with good success include Legionnaires Disease, Toxic Shock Syndrome, Sexually Transmitted Diseases (Syphilis, Gonorrhea, Chlamydia), Smallpox, and Influenza Virus. Of all these, the Tuberculosis model is most applicable to the HIV/AIDS epidemic.

THE U.S. HISTORY OF TUBERCULOSIS

Tuberculosis is a bacteria that initially causes a lung infection. Untreated, it spreads to other parts of the body including the bones, liver, and brain. Like HIV, Tuberculosis bacteria has a unique characteristic in that it changes or mutates in response to single therapy. In the 1950s, researchers and doctors saw drug after drug work and then fail in their patients with Tuberculosis. Even without knowing what we do now about genetics and resistance, intelligent physicians learned to combine their therapies, and then to use triple therapies. Triple therapies, they found, worked superbly.

THE NATIONAL TUBERCULOSIS TREATMENT PROGRAM

At that point, a national treatment program was instituted to provide clear and simple guidelines to all medical personnel on how to treat each case of Tuberculosis, and medications were made available to all people with Tuberculosis. The Public Health System monitored the program. Although Tuberculosis continues to rage worldwide—there are over a billion people infected—the United States has one of the lowest rates in the world. Today more than 60% of the identified cases in the United States each year are in people born in other countries who brought the infection with them to the United States.

The Tuberculosis Treatment Model basically halted new cases in the United States, provided uniform national guidelines on appropriate treatment, got treatment to those infected no matter what their insurance status, reduced the national medical costs due to Tuberculosis, and greatly reduced the deaths due to Tuberculosis. The same could be done for HIV/AIDS.

IT'S TIME FOR AN HIV/AIDS TREATMENT PROGRAM

What allows us to design a successful national program to treat HIV/AIDS now, which could not have been accomplished years before, is our fairly recent breakthrough in understanding how HIV causes damage, and the new developments in therapy that allow us to control this infection in virtually everyone for the first time.

The timing seems right from social and political points of view, as well. Public awareness and compassion are generally sympathetic these days, and a National Treatment Program could be put in place with no or very little new legislation.

ONE MILLION LIVES WILL BE SAVED

I believe a National HIV/AIDS Treatment Program could completely halt the spread of HIV/AIDS in the United States within 18 months, and we've seen the economic savings to be gained—but the most compelling numbers for me are these: **approximately one million lives would be saved over the next 10 years** if we put such a program to work.

FOUR MAJOR COMPONENTS

A National HIV/AIDS Treatment Program would consist of four major components:

- a revised Presidential Commission on HIV/AIDS,
- a limited National Drug Assistance Program,
- access and analysis of all laboratory data on HIV by the Presidential Commission Physician Team,
- public education to encourage voluntary treatment for all people in the United States with HIV infection.

Changes in existing legislation are probably not necessary to institute such a program. A Presidential Commission on HIV/AIDS currently exists.

To institute an effective National Treatment Program, this Commission would need internal reorganization to include:

- a Physician Director - an aggressive, well-trained physician currently practicing HIV clinical medicine,
- six to 12 Regional Physician Directors - chosen by the Physician Director as aggressive practicing HIV clinicians to review and assist in all HIV/AIDS cases in their region,
- appropriate authority - to permit frequent visits by Regional Directors to physicians in their areas to assist in cases,
- appropriate funding - salaries, travel expenses, staff, and equipment for data analysis and tracking by the Commission.

THE GOALS OF THE COMMISSION

The Goals of the Revised Presidential Commission would be to provide **uniform national guidelines** on the treatment of HIV/AIDS within three months consisting of:

- **recommend treatment for all people with HIV/AIDS regardless of T-cell level or HIV viral level,**
- **standardize national therapy as triple therapy to include a powerful protease inhibitor for all cases,**
- **establish a national treatment goal of a zero HIV viral level for all cases.**

If these guidelines are established and followed, we should expect a 75% reduction in pediatric (childhood) HIV/AIDS cases and a 75% reduction in all deaths due to HIV/AIDS within one year, and a 90% reduction in new cases and deaths within two years.

SUMMARY

Current projections are that a person with HIV/AIDS generates $24,000 per year in hospital costs from the date of infection to death. Add to this an additional $10,000 per year in out patient medication, physician, and laboratory, X-ray costs, and a person with HIV/AIDS generates approximately $34,000 in health costs per year. Other costs not included in this estimate include lost income, federal and state support, including SSI and disability payments, and lost tax revenues. The life expectancy of people with HIV/AIDS has been increasing no matter what treatment model is used. Most will live a minimum of 10 years, making the lifetime costs of a person with HIV/AIDS in excess of $340,000.

Early aggressive treatment, is the only model that reduces cost significantly. In providing up front treatment to all people with HIV in the form of triple therapy, many changes to this cost analysis occur:

- hospitalizations costs disappear,
- health is maintained rather than declining,
- disability is avoided. Patients typically lead normal lives and work full-time,
- most Opportunistic Infections are avoided,
- treatment costs for medications are generally fixed at approximately $10,800 per year—or less if block negotiations reduce pharmaceutical costs—as opposed to the current $34,000 per year cost of other, ultimately useless therapies.

The need for a National HIV/AIDS Treatment Program is overwhelming and very much past due. Every day more people are infected with HIV and more people die of HIV/AIDS. In contrast to other important health issues such as heart disease and cancer, HIV/AIDS is an epidemic and continues, as epidemics do, to get worse rather than better. But finally we have the tools to stop the HIV/AIDS epidemic in the United States. I call on the President and the Congress to make it happen.

10
REMISSION & PROGRESS TOWARDS A CURE

10 REMISSION & PROGRESS TOWARDS A CURE

PREDICTING THE FUTURE

Medicines and therapies that we use to treat HIV and other viruses are effective only in **inhibiting** the viruses. They are called **virastatic** medicines. Prior to the 1970s virastatic medicines did not exist and we had nothing to treat viruses at all. We've done very well in a very short time.

What we need to do in the next phase of Clinical Virology is to develop **viracidal** medicines, or viracides. A viracidal medicine would be one that does more than just inhibit, but would lyse, or dissolve and kill a virus as it came in contact with it.

We have already accomplished this for the treatment of bacterial infections. We have medicines that inhibit bacteria, called **bacteriastatic** medicines, like Erythromycin or Tetracycline, used to treat a variety of bacterial infections in humans such as Strept throat, sinus infections, bronchitis, and skin infections. However, they do not kill bacteria directly. We also have developed **bacteriacidal** medicines for this purpose, such as the Penicillin or Keflex. When Penicillin comes in contact with Strept bacteria, it binds to the outer wall of the bacteria and effectively cuts the bacteria open, destroying it. Our next advance in the treatment of HIV and other viruses will likely be the development of medicines or therapies that can destroy viruses safely in the body, thereby clearing the infection quickly and thoroughly.

WHY IS IT SO HARD TO KILL A VIRUS?

After all, heat kills virus. Many solvents also dissolve and kill viruses. The problem is that viruses, unlike bacteria, are structurally very similar to human cells. Viruses contain simple components derived from the human cells that they infect, such as a fat or lipid outer layer, protein inner core, enzymes, and the genetic code of either RNA or DNA. What makes the development of viracidal medicines difficult is that everything developed to date that kills or dissolves HIV and other viruses also kills or dissolves human cells. The key is to find something unique and vulnerable to attack in HIV that is nonexistent or very different in human cells. One must kill HIV without harming the person with HIV.

A second difficulty is that HIV is a retrovirus, replicating in a "retro" or reverse direction, from RNA to DNA, and from there it slips into the human chromosome with help from the HIV enzyme integrase. So even if we could kill all the floating HIV in a person at one time, the "hidden" HIV DNA in the remaining cells would still remain.

The third problem is HIV's constantly changing face. In a person on no treatment, billions of new HIV virions are produced per day with millions of mutations. Thus the therapy must exploit an area of HIV that does not change rapidly, and be able to hit the standard or "wild type" of HIV, as well as millions of mutated forms of HIV—all at one time.

IS A CURE POSSIBLE IN THE NEAR FUTURE?

There are many developments that make the possibility of a cure for HIV likely in the near future. HIV is a new virus in science but it is small compared to most viruses. Its genetic code is one tenth the size of more complex viruses and our understanding of its replication and mutations is comprehensive. Strong social and financial incentives are emerging to find new therapies, vaccines, and a cure.

RESEARCH CONCEPTS THAT MAY LEAD TO A CURE

The development of medicines that kill rather than inhibit HIV replication would make a cure more feasible. These viracides would kill HIV on contact. Therapy might consist of three such medicines given simultaneously over a short period of time to kill all HIV in an infected person. Currently no such viracides exist, although research is moving quickly.

A second approach might be to use current therapy to attain zero viral level for a period exceeding one year to reduce the HIV infection to less than 5% of its original level. Then a therapy or medicine could be given that kills all HIV infected cells throughout the body, including active cells, latent cells, and all reservoirs. At least one medicine is currently undergoing testing that kills HIV infected cells.

A third possible approach might be to develop an external therapy that could be applied to resonate or destroy key structures of the HIV structure. It is not clear that such a therapy is feasible and advances in our knowledge of the resonance of organic molecular structures or subatomic structure would be necessary, as well as advanced applications of Molecular Physics and wave theory. These advances would be difficult but if successful, they could open up entirely new avenues of therapy for all viral diseases—and perhaps in a more mature form, other nonviral diseases, and even cancer.

Thus, there are many areas in science we can now explore in our search for a cure for HIV infection. The problem has been clearly defined. We now need to assign our best scientists and doctors to this urgent problem. The recent appointment of Dr. David Baltimore to direct the development of an HIV vaccine was a major step in the right direction. An equivalent leader needs to be assigned by the federal government to find a cure for this deadly epidemic. I believe that with our recent scientific breakthroughs, a cure could be developed within five years of the start of a "Manhattan" style cure project if the government assigned the most intelligent of our scientists and doctors to work full time and provided rapid and full funding to the effort. It would be costly in the short run, but billions would be saved in the long term.

IN CONCLUSION

HIV IS NOW A TREATABLE DISEASE

The minimum effective therapy for treating HIV is triple therapy. Triple therapy places most people with HIV in Remission. Triple therapy must include three medicines, each of which individually lowers HIV by more than 50%, and preferably by 80% to 90%. In order for this to be possible, the individual's particular strain must be sensitive to each medicine. There can be no resistance as one begins the triple therapy or it will quickly fail. One of the three medicines must be a powerful Protease Inhibitor. *Figure 1* summarizes in schematic form our knowledge of HIV and triple therapy.

GOOD COMPLIANCE IS CRUCIAL

You should not miss any doses if possible and it is most important that by bedtime, every one taking the therapy makes sure he or she has somehow taken the total number of pills required that day. Nucleoside Analogs presently are twice per day and most Protease Inhibitors are three times per day. Future therapies in development such as the Protease Inhibitors AB-378 and 141W94, the Nucleoside Analog 1592 (Abacavir), and the NNRTI DMP-266 will likely be twice per day.

The exact hour one takes these medicines is not as critical. Spreading the doses out during waking hours is probably sufficient.

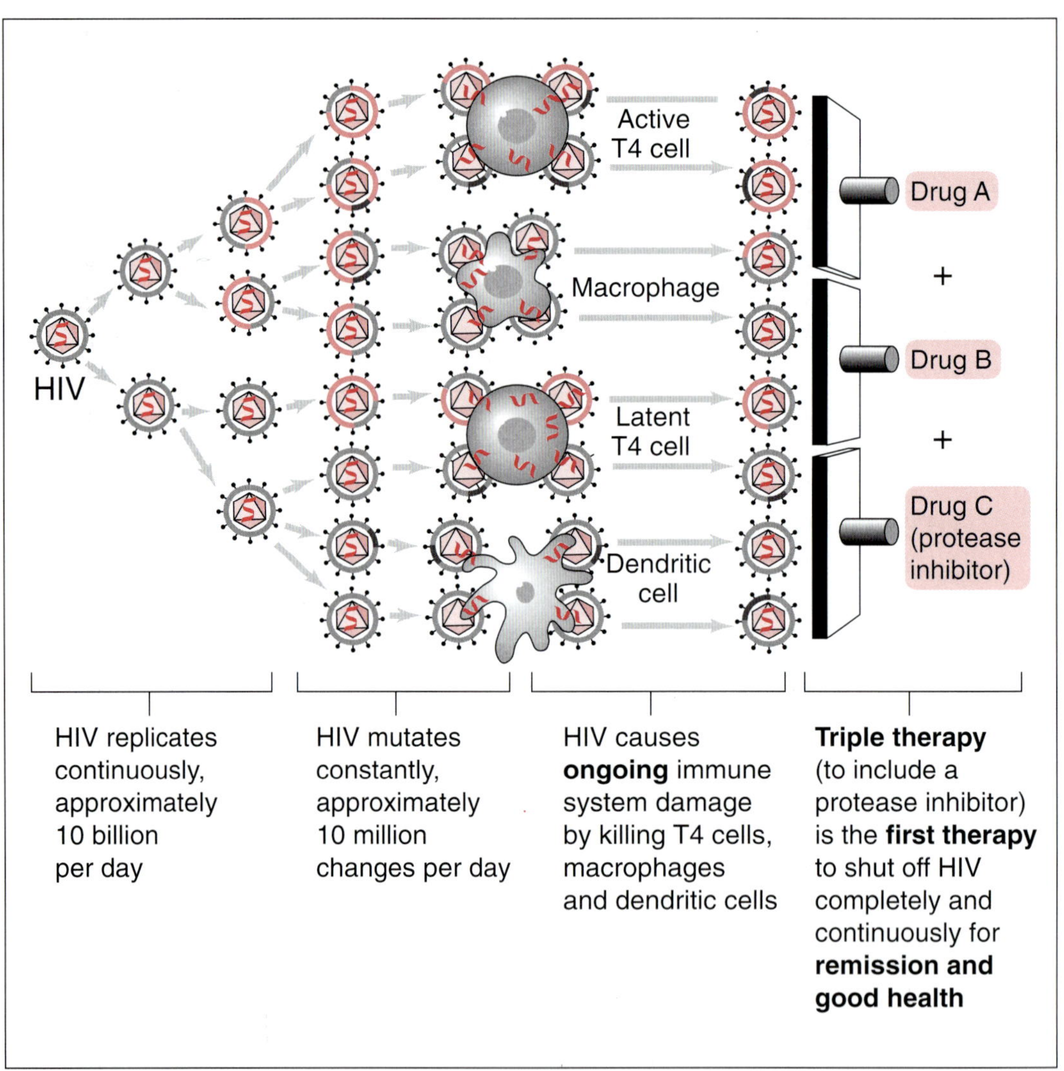

Figure 1 **A summary of our knowledge of HIV and triple therapy: HIV replicates rapidly making many mutational errors. Triple therapy halts replication placing HIV in Remission, halting immune system damage, and restoring health.**

THERE MUST BE NO SIDE EFFECTS

Triple therapy must be free of any significant side effects for each individual. With more than 18 possible triple therapies, there should be a therapy that works and is free of side effects for almost anyone. With a doctor who is experienced and skilled in HIV therapy, and a willing patient, no person with HIV infection need progress to AIDS anymore. The incidence of illness and death is already rapidly dropping. We have the tools and the knowledge right now to place almost everyone with HIV infection in good health and keep them there.

THE MATHEMATICAL MODEL

Dr. David Ho and his research team at the Aaron Diamond Institute in New York have described a two compartment model of HIV, as in Chapter 2, Figure 6.

We have learned that HIV is distributed in two "compartments" or areas of the immune system: more than 95% of HIV is in actively infected T4 cells. The remaining HIV is in the second "compartment" which includes the latent cells, such as the dendritic "relay" cells, of the immune system, the migrating macrophages, the microglial cells of the brain, and latently infected T4 cells.

This picture of the HIV disease process has allowed us to study what types of therapy will work to shut HIV off and why other strategies have failed in the past. HIV produces a huge number of new viruses per day, many of which are mutations. Single therapy fails in this model, as the mutations grow right through individual drugs in weeks to months. This is exactly what we see in clinical or "real" medicine.

Double therapy fails in the model when two simultaneous mutations form a double resistant HIV strain that can grow through two simultaneous medicines. The model predicts this event in approximately three to six months (depending on the drug and the type of mutation required for resistance). In clinical medicine, over the six years I have treated large groups of patients with double therapy (prior to the advent of Protease Inhibitors), double therapies were effective anywhere from six months to two years, which matches the model quite well.

For triple therapy, the model predicts no therapy failure for almost an indefinite period of time, if failure is defined as the occurrence of three separate mutations against three sensitive medicines in a new mutated virus at one time. In other words, it will be very difficult for HIV to mutate through three powerful effective medicines, **if, when starting the triple therapy, all three medicines are working individually.**

Why is this so? It's a matter of odds. The chances of HIV making three specific and simultaneous changes against three effective medicines in a single new virus is exceedingly unlikely. In effect, each medicine in the triple therapy cross protects the other two medicines from resistant strains.

HOW IS TRIPLE THERAPY DOING IN REAL LIFE?

In over one year using triple therapy in my group, I have seen no failure where there was no resistance at the onset, and the patient took the medicines on a daily basis as instructed. In formal studies of triple therapy where all the subjects were drug naive (they had no resistance at the onset), treatment failure has been exceedingly rare. The longest studies have now surpassed two years.

CASE STUDIES

Let's look at a real world example. Here is a random sample of 50 cases under my care that are in Remission. These cases represent the pattern of good response I am seeing in the hundreds of cases under my care. Following are the types of therapy used in these 50 cases:

d4T + 3TC + Crixivan - 48%
AZT + 3TC + Crixivan - 40%
other triple therapies - 6%
quadruple therapy - 6%

The average starting T4 count was 307 with an average improvement of about 160 points during therapy. All cases had an overall improvement in T4 count and clinical health, with some T4 count increases exceeding 400 points. Those with starting T4 counts less than 100 appeared to improve more slowly than those with starting T4 counts above 100. Some cases with lower T4 counts took six months or more to move above 100, but all improved.

The average starting HIV viral level was 80,000 copies/ml and one case began with viral levels exceeding 1.2 million. There appeared to be no difference in the rate of decline of HIV based on the starting HIV level—both those with high viral levels and low viral levels responded rapidly to therapy. Those cases that took the longest to reach undetectable again were generally those patients with starting T4 counts below 100 cells/ml.

Health improvements were dramatic and sustained. One patient who came to me initially with a T4 count of less than 50 cells and a viral level above one million, was found to have concurrent Cryptococcal pneumonia, and early CMV and MAI. After two months of triple therapy and treatment for his infections, his HIV level decreased to less than 20 copies per ml and his T4 count slowly rose to 150, then 300, then to 450. His infections resolved and he is now in normal health.

Another patient with long standing CMV retinitis requiring intravenous Ganciclovir, Foscarnet, and intraocular implants also had resistant candidiasis and recurrent Pseudomonas pneumonia. On effective HIV therapy, he is in Remission, off intravenous medicines, has almost normal eyesight, and has returned to the gym and part-time work. His T4 count has increased more than 150 points and is stable.

One patient who had a sustained zero T4 count, had a T4 recovery on effective therapy from zero to 10, then 20, then 40, then 80, then 150, and then slowly increased above 300, with corresponding global improvements in energy and weight, and resolution of chronic skin problems and bronchitis.

Three cases of extensive skin, lung, and limb Kaposi's Sarcoma stabilized or resolved with concurrent brief radiation in one case, and limited cycles of Doxil therapy in two other cases.

Side effects from therapy were rare, not exceeding 10%, with none being serious. Most patients achieved Remission without side effects or problems by the first or second selection of triple therapy and reached an undetectable HIV viral level by month two or three on average.

These 50 cases have remained in Remission an average of six months and are continuing. Some have been in Remission for a year or more.

FOUR DRUG THERAPY

In approximately 5% of cases, HIV viral levels do not quite reduce to undetectable on triple therapy. Most of these cases are among people with very advanced HIV infection, for instance with a T4 count less than 100, an HIV level exceeding 100,000 to one million, and in those who have taken multiple prior medicines and likely have a multi-resistant HIV strain. Part of the solution is to determine the sensitive (effective) medicines by Comparison PCR or if available, an accurate HIV Sensitivity Assay. We may be able to reduce such a person's HIV level well below 10,000 on triple therapy, but occasionally need a fourth medicine to reach zero. The addition of ddI, 3TC, or a second Protease Inhibitor may be helpful in difficult cases, and the addition of either 1592 or DMP-266 or their combination may be available in the near future. Four-drug therapy is not often necessary, but the goal is an undetectable or zero viral level, and the point is to achieve that goal in every case, whatever it takes.

FREQUENT ERRORS ARE BEING MADE

However, many researchers and many doctors are making frequent mistakes. One recent report was about a triple therapy study of AZT + 3TC + Crixivan, in people who had been on AZT for six months or more. It is highly likely that many of these people are resistant to AZT, as there is at least 60% resistance at one year of single therapy AZT. Some reports indicate that 3TC "reverses" AZT resistance, but newer studies indicate this phenomenon is less common than previously reported. To their dismay researchers have had to report 20% failure in the AZT + 3TC + Crixivan study using people previously on AZT single therapy.

They're lucky their treatment failure wasn't greater than 20% because they used individuals in the study who were resistant to AZT. Had they tested AZT resistance or switched the entire group to d4T + 3TC + Crixivan, so that all three medicines were working at the onset, they would not likely see any treatment failure at all. **For a triple therapy to work long term, no resistance may exist in any of the individual medicines when the person first starts therapy.**

ACHIEVING AND MAINTAINING REMISSION

The Two Compartment Model of HIV viral dynamics has not only shown us how to approach therapy, it has predicted that as we initiate triple therapy, HIV will be rapidly cleared from the T4 cells and slowly cleared from the latent cells. With the declining HIV infection, the damage to the immune system stops, and we see a two phase slightly delayed increase in T4 count and a dramatic, sustained global improvement in the person's health.

In fact, most people return to normal health and remain in normal health as long as they continue to take their medicines and maintain their Remission. In Remission, with undetectable viral levels, HIV declines rapidly in the blood, and to our surprise, throughout the body. Multiple tissue studies of people in Remission show that HIV is undetectable in lymph nodes, gastrointestinal tissue, blood, semen, and even the spinal fluid after one to two years of effective triple therapy.

It appears that effective triple therapy with Remission allows the body to clear up to 95% or more of HIV out of the body over a period of one to two years. What remains is a small amount of integrated or proviral DNA which we have not yet discovered how to eliminate, meaning that triple therapy must be continued for the indefinite future or the HIV infection will return and begin the cycle of damage once again.

Preliminary studies of damaged lymph node and other immune system tissue of those people in Remission on triple therapy demonstrate areas of new growing immune tissue where previously there was damaged tissue full of virus. Although this is very preliminary, it means that the body may actually be able to repair the damaged immune system on its own, if we can keep HIV completely and continuously shut off by effective triple therapy.

PREVENTING INFECTIONS

Opportunistic Infections are preventable in people with HIV. A simple 3 - 2 - 1 algorithm recommends protection when one's T4 counts reach 300, 200, and 100, as follows:

T4 less than	Infection risk	Prevention
300	PCP	Septra or Dapsone
200	Crypto, Candida	Fluconazole
100	MAI	Azithromycin or Biaxin
	Toxo	Septra or Azithromycin
	CMV	if culture +, Ganciclovir
all	Zoster, Herpes	Acyclovir

One could do less, perhaps wait to prophylax against PCP when the T4 level drops below 200, but some cases would be missed. My approach is to prevent all Opportunistic Infections if possible.

It is now known that when a person with HIV has an Opportunistic Infection, their HIV viral levels soar dangerously high, many times exceeding one million copies per milliliter. This large coactivation of HIV infection during an Opportunistic Infection leads to rapid immune system damage, emergence of multi-resistant HIV strains, and treatment failure. For this reason, we should renew our efforts to prevent all serious infections in people with HIV.

New research also indicates that the daily use of Acyclovir reduces the occurrence of lymphoma in people with HIV by as much as 80%. This is not unexpected as most lymphomas in HIV are caused by a Herpes virus called Epstein Barr, which is suppressed by the use of Acyclovir. Thus Acyclovir has a multiple role in preventing the Opportunistic Infections of Herpes and Zoster, and dramatically reducing the risk of lymphoma.

After effective triple therapy is begun and the HIV viral level is maintained at zero, and one's T4 count rises to higher levels and remains there for more than one month, I recommend the prevention strategy be reassessed based on the new level. Many times some of the prophylactic medicines can be safely eliminated. However, if any active Opportunistic Infections occur in the course of treatment, a more cautious approach may be necessary, which is an area of ongoing research in many academic centers nationwide.

WASTING SYNDROME IS REVERSIBLE

Wasting Syndrome is common and its cause is relatively easy to identify and treat. It is usually caused by a new medical problem, such as an infection, diarrhea syndrome, or tumor, a lack of sufficient calorie intake, or a hormone deficiency. Testosterone deficiency is quite common at T4 counts below 300 in men, probably a result of direct damage of HIV to the gonads, although it is unknown if some of the medicines are also diminishing gonadal function. Treatment is with replacement testosterone. A form of synthetic testosterone, Nandrolone, is FDA approved, low cost, and may be used alone or with testosterone therapy for two to four months, or as necessary, to encourage weight gain. No cases of Wasting Syndrome should go untreated, and in my experience they are all quite solvable.

FINALLY

Resistant medicines are still a large unidentified problem in HIV treatment and in my experience are one of the major causes of treatment failure, in addition to poor compliance with medicines. Resistance can be identified and avoided. Today we have at least one HIV sensitivity test available, the HIV-1 GenotypeR and we can also test for resistance using Comparison PCR. Our next generation of tests of HIV sensitivity should make resistance even easier to identify, but any test is only as good as the doctor who administers it and monitors it and the patient who is also an active participant in the therapy.

The field of HIV has advanced rapidly and is continuing to advance further. Effective triple therapy is now available to place HIV and AIDS in Remission, and in doing so, restores good health. Infections can be prevented and Wasting Syndrome reversed. With knowledge and understanding, the hope for a long life and even for a cure in the near future is becoming a reality.

APPENDIX

Your Medicine Sheet

Name:__________________ Allergies:__________________

Anti-HIV Medicines

Name	Dose	How many	How often	Notes:

Prevention Medicines

Name	Dose	How many	How often	Notes:

Other Medicines

Name	Dose	How many	How often	Notes:

A-1 **The medicines currently taken by a person with HIV are written on the Medication Sheet.** The Medication Sheet is divided into three sections: for HIV medicines (AZT, d4T, Crixivan, Nelfinavir), for medicines to prevent infection (Septra/Bactrim, Fluconazole, Azithromycin), and for other medicines (Testosterone, Clariton, etc.). When therapy is changed, the old Medication Sheet is filed or discarded and a new one written.

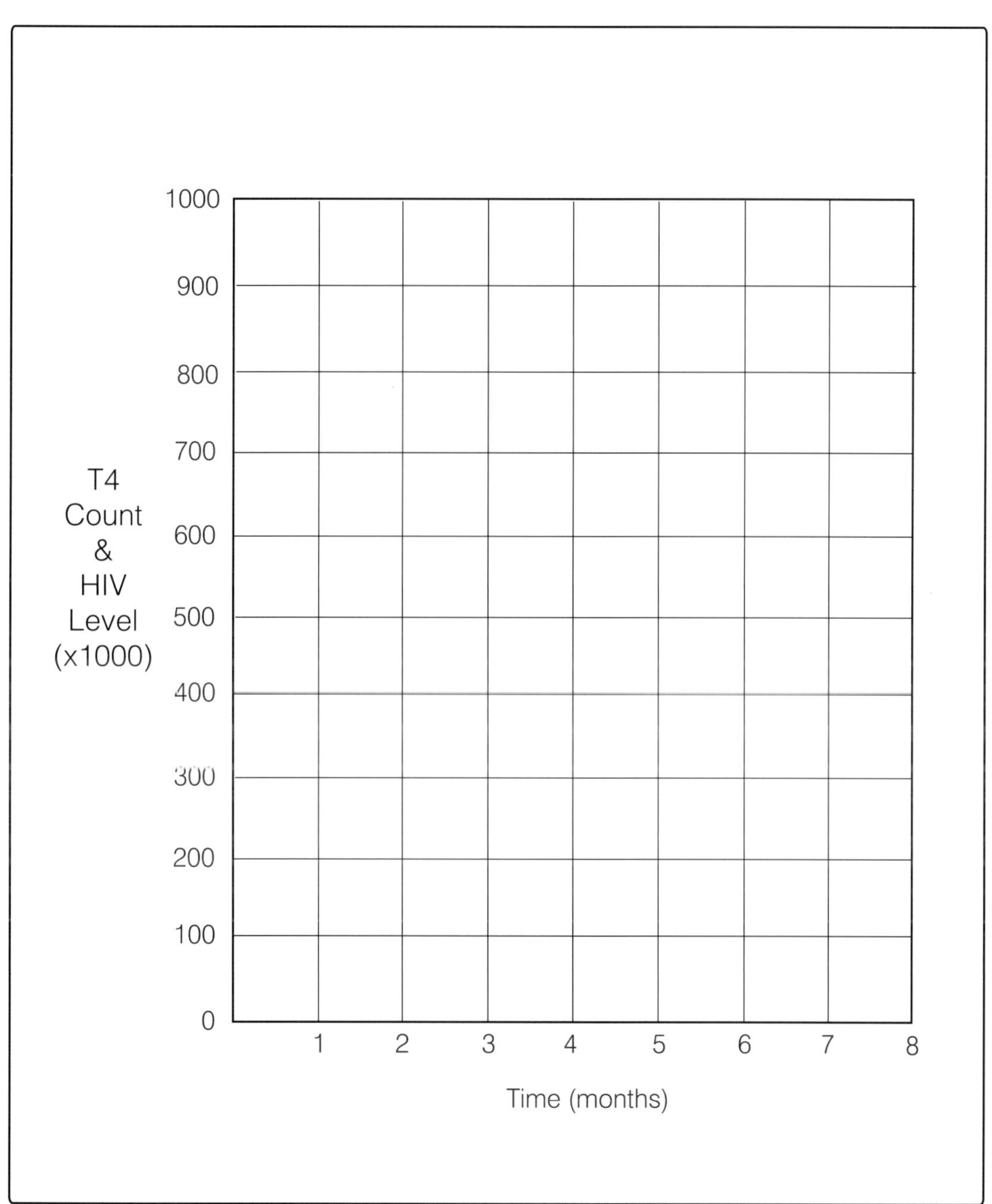

A-2 **Lab results are graphed on the T4/HIV graph each time they are done.** The T4 count measures the strength of the immune system and is graphed using a solid line with dots as data points. The HIV viral level (PCR or b-DNA) measures the activity of HIV infection and is graphed using a solid line with circles around dots for data points. For HIV level, data is graphed in thousands. In other words, an HIV level of 120,000 is graphed as 120k, where k = 1000.

REFERENCES

1. Barre-Sinoussi F, et al: Isolation of a T-lymphotropic retrovirus from a patient at risk for AIDS. Science 1983;220:868-871
2. Centers for Disease Control: U.S. HIV and AIDS cases reported through December 1996. HIV/AIDS Surveillance Report. 1996;8:1-39
3. Torres R, et al: Impact of potent new antiretroviral therapies on in-patient and outpatient hospital utilization by HIV-infected persons. [Abstract 264], 4th Conference on Retroviruses and Opportunistic Infections, Washington, D.C., 1997
4. Scofield, CI, et al: The Holy Bible. New York, Oxford University Press, 1945
5. Williams G, et al: AIDS in 1959? Lancet 1983;2:1136
6. Williams G, et al: Cytomegalic inclusion disease and pneumocystis carinii infection in an adult. Lancet 1960;ii:951-955
7. Witte MH, et al: AIDS in 1968. JAMA 1984;251:2657.
8. Elvin-Lewis M, et al: Systemic chlamydial infection associated with generalized lymphedema and lymphangiosarcoma. Lymphology 1073;6:113-121
9. Nahmias AJ, et al: Evidence for human infection with an HTLV III/LAV like virus in central Africa, 1959. Lancet 1986:1250-1252
10. Brunet JB, et al: AIDS in France. Lancet 1983:700-701
11. Clumeck N, et al: AIDS in black Africans. Lancet 1983:642
12. Quinn TC, et al: AIDS in Africa: an epidemiologic paradigm. Science 1986;234:955-963
13. Schapiro R, et al: Early AIDS case discovered. The New Physician 1987;36:12
14. Knox RA: Study in Zaire shows AIDS may have existed for 100 years. Boston Globe 1988 Feb 6;6
15. Shilts R: What Africa's AIDS epidemic reveals. San Francisco Chronicle 1987 June 8;4
16. Shilts R: And the Band Played On. New York, St Martin's Press, 1987
17. Garrett L: The Coming Plague. New York, Penguin Books, 1994
18. Auerbach DM, et al: Epidemiologic aspects of the current outbreak of kaposi's sarcoma and opportunistic infections. N Engl J Med 1982;306:248-252
19. Gottlieb MS, et al: Pneumocystis pneumonia-LosAngeles. MMWR 1981;30:250-252

20. Gallo RC, et al: Isolation of a T-Lymphotropic retrovirus from a patient at risk for AIDS. Science 1983;220:865-867
21. Task Force on AIDS, CDC: Update on acquired immune deficiency syndrome (AIDS) -United States. MMWR 1982;31:507-514
22. Committee on a National Strategy for AIDS, National Academy of Sciences: Confronting AIDS: Directions for Public Health, Health Care, and Research. Washington D.C., National Academy Press, 1986
23. Kanki PJ, et al: Isolation of T-lymphotropic Retrovirus related to HTLV-III/LAV from wild-caught African green monkeys. Science 1985;230:951-954
24. Brunet JB, et al: The international occurrence of AIDS. Ann Intern Med 1985;103:670-674
25. Rutherford GW: Statistics from SF department of public health. AIDS File, San Francisco General Hospital Medical Center 1986 Jan;1:3
26. Pape JW: The acquired immunodeficiency syndrome in Haiti. Ann Intern Med 1985;103:674-678
27. Safai B, et al: The natural history of kaposi's sarcoma in acquired immunodeficiency syndrome. Ann Intern Med 1985;103:744-750
28. Task force on kapos's sarcoma and opportunistic infections, CDC;Update on kaposi's sarcoma and opportunistic Infections in previously healthy persons-United States. MMWR 1982;31:294-301
29. Brunet JB, et al: Update: acquired immunodeficiency syndrome-Europe. MMWR 1985;34:583-589
30. Albert J, et al: A new human retrovirus isolate of west African origin (SBL-6669) and its relationship to HTLV-IV, LAV-II, and HTLV-IIIB. AIDS Res Hum Retroviruses 1987;3:3-10
31. DeVita VT, Jr., et al: AIDS: Etiology, Diagnosis, Treatment, and Prevention. Philadelphia, JB Lippincott Company, 1985
32. Wong-Staal F, et al: Molecular biology of human T-lymphotropic retroviruses. Cancer Res (suppl) 1985;45:4539s-4544s
33. Essex M, et al: Retroviruses associated with leukemia and ablative syndromes in animals and in human beings. Cancer Res (suppl) 1985;45:4534s-4538s
34. Sullivan R: AIDS-related virus is found in Africa. New York Times 1987 June 2;19,23
35. Verones R: HIV-2 in Brazil. Lancet 1987;2:402
36. Senechek DR: Lymphadenopathy and AIDS. Boston, Harvard/HST Thesis, 1988

37. Piot P: HIV/AIDS: The global status and response to the epidemic. [Abstract S2], the 4th Conference on Retroviruses and Opportunistic Infections, Washington D.C., 23 Jan 1997
38. Koop CE: Surgeon general's report on AIDS. U.S. Department of Health and Human Services 1986 Oct
39. Gelmann EP, et al: Proviral DNA of a retrovirus, human T-cell leukemia virus, in two patients with AIDS. Science 1983;220:862-864
40. Fields BN, et al: Virology. New York, Raven Press, 1985
41. Seligmann M, et al: Immunology of human immunodeficiency virus infection and the acquired immunodeficiency syndrome. Ann Intern Med 1987;107:234-242
42. Van de Graff M, et al: Transmission of human immunodeficiency virus (HIV/HTLV-III/LAV): a review. Infection 1986;14:203-211
43. Peterman TA, et al: Sexual transmission of human immunodeficiency virus. JAMA 1986;256:2222-2226
44. Chamberland ME, et al: Heterosexually acquired infection with human immunodeficiency virus (HIV). Ann Intern Med 1987;107:763-766
45. Shilts R: Uganda in desperate pursuit of runaway AIDS. San Francisco Chronicle 1987 Oct 6:A8-9
46. Baetz-Greenwalt B: AIDS in infants and children. New Physician 1987:33-36
47. Jaffee HW, et al: Lack of HIV transmission in the practice of a dentist with AIDS. Ann Intern Med 1994;121:855-859
48. Villee CA: Biology. WB Saunders Company, Philadelphia, 1977
49. Gallo RC, et al: A human T-lymphotropic retrovirus (HTLV-III) as the cause of the acquired immunodeficiency syndrome. Ann Intern Med 1985;103:679-689
50. Montagnier L: Lymphadenopathy-associated virus: from molecular biology to pathogenicity. Ann Intern Med 1985;103:689-693
51. Levy JA, et al: Infection by the retrovirus associated with the acquired immunodeficiency syndrome. Ann Intern Med 1985;103:694-699
52. Stringfellow DA, et al: Virology. Michigan, Upjohn, 1983
53. Hoxie JA: Current concepts in virology of infection with human immunodeficiency virus (HIV): a view from the III International Conference on AIDS. Ann Intern Med 1987 ;107:406-408
54. McCutchan FE: HIV genetic diversity. [Abstract Mo.02:2], the XI International Conference on AIDS. Vancouver 1996
55. Starcich B, et al: Characterization of long terminal repeat sequences of HTLV-III. Science 1985;227:538-540
56. Ratner L, et al: Complete nucleotide sequence of the AIDS virus, HTLV-III. Nature 1985;313:277-284

57. Essex M, et al: Antigens of human T-lymphotropic virus type III/lymphadenopathy associated virus. Ann Intern Med 1985;103:700-703
58. Wong-Staal F, et al: Human immunodeficiency virus: the eighth gene. AIDS Res Hum Retroviruses 1987;3:33-39
59. Ratner L, et al: Complete nucleotide sequences of functional clones of the AIDS virus. AIDS Res Hum Retroviruses 1987;3:57-69
60. Sodroski J: Human retroviruses: HTLV I, II, III. [class notes], Harvard Medical School Course in Microbiology 1985 Dec
61. Grant I, et al: Evidence for early CNS involvement in AIDS and other human immunodeficiency virus (HIV) infections. Ann Intern Med 1987;107:828-836
62. Ho DD: Can HIV be eradicated from an infected person? [Abstract S1], 4th Conference on Retroviruses and Opportunistic Infections, Washington D.C., 1997
63. Perelson A: Viral and cellular dynamics implications for antiretroviral therapy. [Abstract L1], 4th Conference on Retroviruses and Opportunistic Infections, Washington D.C., 1997
64. Baggiolini M: Chemokines: structures and biological activities. [Abstract L2], 4th Conference on Retroviruses and Opportunistic Infections, Washington D.C., 1997
65. Sodroski J: Viral and Host Factors in HIV Entry. [Abstract S8], 4th Conference on Retroviruses and Opportunistic Infections, Washington D.C., 1997
66. Landau N: The role of CCR-5 in HIV entry and susceptibility of individuals to infection. [Abstract S11], 4th Conference on Retroviurses and Opportunistic Infections, Washington D.C., 1997
67. Meyer PR, et al: An immunopathologic evaluation of lymph nodes from monkey and man with acquired immune deficiency syndromes and related conditions. Hem Oncology Jul-Sep;3:199-210
68. Tenner-Raczk K, et al: HTLV-III/LAV viral antigens in lymph nodes of homosexual men with persistent generalized lymphadenopathy and AIDS. Amer J Path 1986;123:9-15
69. Anderson MG, et al: Persistent lymphadenopathy in homosexual men: a clinical and ultrastructural study. Lancet 198424:880-2.
70. Humphrey JH: Virus-like particles in AIDS-related lymphadenopathy. Lancet 1984;2:643
71. Koenig S, et al: immunology of infection with the human immunodeficiency virus (HIV); a view from the III International Conference on AIDS. Ann Intern Med 1987;107:409-411

72. Bowen DL, et al: Immunopathogenesis of the acquired immunodeficiency syndrome. Ann Intern Med 1985;103:704-709
73. Seligmann M, et al: Immunology of human immunodeficiency virus infection and the acquired immunodeficiency syndrome. Ann Intern Med 1987;107:234-242
74. Boyko WJ, et al: The Vancouver lymphadenopathy-AIDS study 3. relation of HTLV-III seropositivity, immune status and lymphadenopathy. Can Med Assoc J 1985;133:28-32
75. Eyster ME, et al: Natural history of human immunodeficiency virus infections in hemophiliacs: effects of T cell subsets, platelet counts, and age. Ann Intern Med 1987;107:1-6
76. Goedert JJ, et al: Effect of T4 count and cofactors on the incidence of AIDS in homosexual men infected with human immunodeficiency virus. JAMA 1987;257:331-334
77. Grody WW, et al: Thymus involution in the acquired immunodeficiency syndrome. Amer J Clin Path 1985;84:85-95
78. Abrams DI, et al: AIDS-related benign lymphadenopathy and malignant lymphoma: clinical aspects and virologic interactions. AIDS Res 1986 (suppl 1);2:S131-S140
79. Cooper DA, et al: Acute AIDS retrovirus infection. Lancet 1985:537-540
80. Calabrese LH, et al: Acute infection with the human immunodeficiency virus (HIV) associated with acute brachial neuritis and exanthematous rash. Ann Intern Med 1987;107:849-851
81. Rustin MHA, et al: The acute exanthem associated with seroconversion to human T-cell lymphotrophic virus III in a homosexual man. J Infec 1986;12:161-163
82. Ho DD, et al: Primary human T-lymphotropic virus type III infection. Ann Intern Med 1985;103:880-883
83. Schacker T, et al: Clinical and epidemiologic features of primary HIV infection. Ann Intern Med 1996;125:257-264
84. Carne CA, et al: Acute encephalopathy coincident with seroconversion for anti-HTLV-III. Lancet 1985 Nov 30:1206-1208
85. Volberding PA: The clinical spectrum of the acquired immunodeficiency syndrome: implications for comprehensive patient care. Ann Intern Med 1985;103:729-733
86. Kaslow RA, et al: Infection with the human immunodeficiency virus: clinical manifestations and their relationship to immune deficiency. Ann Intern Med 1987;107:474-480
87. Kaplan JE, et al: Lymphadenopathy syndrome in homosexual men. JAMA 1987;257:335-339

88. CDC, U.S. Department of Health and Human Services: Classification system for human T-lymphotropic virus type III/lymphadenopathy-associated virus infections. Ann Intern Med 1986;105:234-237
89. CDC: Revision of the CDC surveillance case definition for AIDS. JAMA 1987;258:1143-1145, 1149, 1153-54
90. CDC:1993 revised classification system for HIV infection and expanded surveillance case definition for AIDS among adolescents and adults. MMWR 1992;41(No. RR-17)
91. Mellors JW, et al: Quantitation of HIV-1 RNA in plasma predicts outcome after seroconversion. Ann Intern Med 1995;122:573-579
92. Mellors JW, et al: Viral load: better predictor of HIV disease progression and survival (reported through HIV Information Network 11 Feb 1996), [Abstract 251], 3rd Conference on Retroviruses and Opportunistic Infections, 1996
93. Collier A: In with the new: how will the new drugs be used? [Abstract S52], 4th Conference on Retroviruses and Opportunistic Infections, Washington, D.C., 1997
94. GlaxoWellcome: Retrovir (zidovudine) capsules and syrup. Package insert. Feb 1996.
95. Bristol-Myers Squibb: Zerit (stavudine) capsules. Package insert with revision. Jan 1996
96. Bristol-Myers Squibb: Videx (didanosine). Package insert with revision. Feb 1996
97. Roche Laboratories: Hivid (Zalcitabine). Package insert with revision. July 1996
98. GlaxoWellcome: Epivir tablets and solution (lamivudine). Package insert. Jan 1996
99. Prasad VR: Mutations associated with 3TC-resistance enhance the polymerase fidelity of HIV-1 RT. [Abstract Mo.A.381], XI International Conference on AIDS, Vancouver, 1996
100. Harrigan R, et al: Antiretroviral activity and resistance profile of the carbocyclic nucleoside HIV reverse transcriptase inhibitor 1592U89. [Abstract 15], 4th Conference on Retroviruses and Opportunistic Infections, Washington, D.C., 1997
101. Project Inform: Protease Inhibitors: Choices and Analysis. PI Perspective. 1996;18:1-5
102. Project Inform: Update on Protease Inhibitors. PI Perspective 1996;18:1-4
103. Roche Laboratories: Invirase (Saquinavir mesylate). Package insert with revision. June 1996

104. Schapiro JM, et al: The effect of high-dose saquinavir on viral load and CD4+ T-cell counts in HIV-infected patients. Ann Intern Med. 1996;124:1039-50
105. Merck & Co: Crixivan (indivavir sulfate). Package insert. March 1996
106. Abbott Laboratories: Norvir (ritonavir capsules/oral solution). Package insert with revision. Nov 1996; Ref. 03-4720-R3
107. Markowitz M, et al: A preliminary study of Ritonavir, an inhibitor of HIV-1 protease, to treat HIV-1 infection. N Eng J Med. 1995;333:1534-1540
108. Agouron Pharmaceuticals: Viracept (nelfinavir mesylate). Package insert with revision. March 1997
109. Roxane Labs: Viramune (nevirapine). Package insert. 1997
110. Pharmacia & Upjohn: Rescriptor (delavirdine mesylate tablets). Package insert. 1997
111. Freimuth WW, et al: Delavirdine (DLV) combined with zidovudine (ZDV) or didanosine (ddI) produces sustained reduction in viral burden and increases in CD4 count in early and advanced HIV-1 infection. [Abstract Mo.B.295], XI International Conference on AIDS. Vancouver 1996
112. Wathen LK, et al: Phenotypic sensitivity of HIV-1 viral isolates during combination delavirdine + zidovudine therapy. [Abstract 12], 4th Conference on Retroviruses and Opportunistic Infections, Washington, D.C., 1997
113. FaxWatch: Product News: Aronex Pharmaceuticals/Zintevir. HIV Update. 18 Nov 1996
114. Cooper D, et al: the CAESAR trial: final results. [Abstract 367], 4th Conference on Retreviruses and Opportunistic Infection, Washington, D.C., 1997
115. Rozenbaum W, the AVANTI Study Group: a randomised, double blind, comparative trial to evaluate the efficacy, safety, and tolerance of combination antiretroviral regimens for the treatment of HIV-1 infection: AZT/3TC vs. AZT/3TC/loviride in anti-retroviral naive patients. [Abstract 368], 4th Conference on Retroviruses and Opportunistic Infections, Washington, D.C., 1997
116. Sham H, et al: Design, synthesis and biological properties of ABT-378, a highly potent HIV protease inhibitor. [Abstract 14], 4th Conference on Retroviruses and Opportunistic Infections, Washington, D.C., 1997
117. Schooley RT, et al: Preliminary data from a phase I/II study on the safety and antiviral efficacy of the combination of 141W94 plus 1592U89 in HIV-infected patients with 150 to 400 CD4+ cells/mm3. [Abstract LB3], 4th Conference on Retroviruses and Opportunistic Infections, 1997

118. Moxham CP, et al: Preliminary efficacy and safety of repeated multiple doses of MKC-442 in HIV-infected volunteers. [Abstract LBI], 4th Conference on Retroviruses and Opportunistic Infections, Washington, D.C., 1997
119. Ruiz N, et al: A double-blind pilot study to evaluate the antiretroviral activity, tolerability of DMP-266 in combination with indinavir. [Abstract LB2], 4th Conference on Retroviruses and Opportunistic Infections, Washington, D.C., 1997
120. Young SD: L-743,726 (DMP-266): a novel, highly potent nonnucleoside inhibitor of HIV-1 reverse transcriptase. [Abstract Mo.A.1077], XI International Conference on AIDS, Vancouver 1996
121. Carpenter CCJ, et al: Antiretroviral therapy for HIV Infection in 1996: recommendations of an international panel. JAMA 1996;276:146-154
122. Sande MA, et al: Antiretroviral therapy in adult HIV-infected patients: recommendations from a state-of-the-art conference. JAMA 1993;270:2583-2589
123. Hammer S: Advances in antiretroviral therapy and viral load monitoring. [Abstract Mo.01], XI International Conference on AIDS, Vancouver 1996
124. Brun-Vezinet F, et al: HIV viral load changes in Delta patients. [Abstract Mo.B.292], XI International Conference on AIDS , Vancouver 1996
125. Katzenstein DA, et al: Suppression of plasma HIV RNA by RT inhibitors prevents AIDS and death in ACTG 175: combination and monotherapy with ZDV, ddI, and ddC. [Abstract Mo.B.293], XI International Conference on AIDS, Vancouver 1996
126. Cavert W, et al: Quantitative in situ hybridization (ISH) measurement of HIV-1 RNA clearance kinetics from lymphoid tissue (LT) cellular compartments during triple-drug therapy [Abstract LB9], 4th Conference on Retroviruses and Opportunistic Infections, Washington, D.C., 1997
127. Wong JK, et al: Reduction of HIV in blood and lymph nodes after potent antiretroviral therpy [Abstract LB10], 4th Conference on Retroviruses and Opportunistic Infections, Washington, D.C., 1997
128. Kotler DP, et al: Effect of combination antiretroviral therapy upon mucosal viral RNA burden and apoptosis [Abstract LB11], 4th Conference on Retroviruses and Opportunistic Infections, Washington, D.C., 1997
129. Havlir DV, et al: Viral dynamics of HIV: implications for drug development and therapeutic strategies. Ann Intern Med. 1996;124:984-994
130. Saag MS, et al: HIV viral load markers in clinical practice. Nat Med.1996;2:625-629

131. Palenicek JP, et al: Weight loss prior to clinical AIDS as a predictor of survival. Multicenter AIDS Cohort Study Investigators. J AIDS Hum Retrovirol. 1996;10:366-373
132. Suttmann U, et al: Incidence and prognostic value of malnutrition and wasting in human immunodeficiency virus-infected outpatients. J AIDS Hum Retrovirol. 1995;8:239-246
133. Ott M, et al: Bioelectrical impedance analysis as a predictor of survival in patients with human immunodeficiency virus infection. J AIDS Hum Retrovirol. 1995;9:20-25
134. Kotler DP, et al: Magnitude of body-cell-mass depletion and the timing of death from wasting in AIDS. Am J Clin Nutr. 1989;50:444-447
135. Guenter P, et al: Relationships among nutritional status, disease progression, and survival in HIV infection. J AIDS 1993;6:1130-1138
136. Kotler DP, et al: Enteral alimentation and repletion of body cell mass in malnourished patients with acquired immunodeficeincy syndrome. AM J Clin Nutr. 1991;53:149-154
137. Kotler DP, et al: Effect of home total parenteral nutrition on body composition in patients with acquired immunodeficiency syndrome. J Parenter Enteral Nutr. 1990;14:454-458
138. Von Roenn JH, et al: Megestrol acetate in patients with AIDS-related cachexia. Ann Intern Med. 1994;121:393-399
139. Oster MH, et al: Megestrol acetate in patients with AIDS and cachexia. Ann Intern Med. 1994;121:400-408
140. Waters D, et al: Recombinant human growth hormone, insulin-like growth factor 1, and combination therapy in AIDS-associated wasting. Ann Intern Med. 1996;125:865-872
141. Schambelan M, et al: Recombinant human growth hormone in patients with HIV-associated wasting. Ann Intern Med. 1996;125:873-882
142. Wilcox CM, et al: Esophageal ulceration in human immunodeficiency virus infection: causes, response to therapy, and long-term outcome. Ann Intern Med. 1995;123:143-149
143. Edwards P, et al: Esophageal ulceration induced by zidovudine. Ann Intern Med. 1990;112:65-66
144. Indorf AS, et al: Esophageal ulceration induced by zalcitabine (ddC). Ann Intern Med. 1992;117:133-134
145. Bucher G, et al: A prospective study on the safety and effect of nandrolone decanoate in HIV-positive patients. [Abstract Mo.B.423], XI International Conference on AIDS, Vancouver 1996

146. Rabkin JG et al: Treatment of depression in HIV+ men: literature review and report of an ongoing study of testosterone replacement therapy. [abstract pending publication]. 1996:1-2
147. Rabkin JG, et al: Testosterone replacement therapy in HIV illness. Gen Hosp Psychiatry 1995;17:37-42
148. Leinung MC, et al: Induction of adrenal suppression by megestrol acetate in patients with AIDS. Ann Intern Med. 1995;122:843-845
149. Dieterich DT: Advances in the pathophysiology and treatment of HIV-associated wasting. Improving the Management of HIV Disease (International AIDS Society-USA). 1997;4:24-27
150. Masur H, et al: CD4 counts as predictors of opportunistic pneumonias in HIV infection. Ann Intern Med. 1989;111:223-231
151. Moore RD, et al: Natural history of opportunistic disease in an HIV-infected urban clinical cohort. Ann Intern Med. 1996;124:633-642
152. Members of the USPHS/IDSA prevention of opportunistic infections working group: USPHS/IDSA guidelines for the prevention of opportunistic infections in persons infected with HIV: a summary. Ann Intern Med. 1996;124:348-368
153. Powderly WG: Prophylaxis for HIV-related infections: a work in progress. Ann Intern Med. 1996;124:342-344
154. Bozzette SA, et al: A randomized trial of three antipneumocystis agents in patients with advanced human immunodeficiency virus infection. N Engl J Med. 1995;332:693-699
155. Saah AJ, et al: Predictors for failure of Pneumocystis carinii pneumonia prophylaxis. Multicenter AIDS Cohort Study. JAMA. 1995;273:1197-1202
156. Nelson MR, et al: The role of azoles in the treatment and prophylaxis of cryptococcal disease in HIV infection. AIDS. 1994;8:651-654
157. Powderly WG, et al: A randomized trial comparing fluconazole with clotrimazole troches for the prevention of fungal infections in patients with advanced human immunodeficiency virus infection. N Engl J Med. 1995;332:700-705
158. Parente F, et al: Prevention of symptomatic recurrences of esophageal candidiasis in AIDS patients after the first episode: a prospective open study. Am J Gastroenterol. 1994;89:416-420
159. Selik RM, et al: Trends in infectious diseases and cancers among persons dying of HIV infection in the United States from 1987 to 1992. Ann Intern Med. 1995;123:933-936
160. Schneider MM, et al: Efficacy and toxicity of two doses of trimethoprim-sulfamethoxazole as primary prophylaxis against

pneumocystis carinii pneumonia in patients with human immunodeficiency virus. J Infect Dis. 1995;171:1632-1636

161. Podzamczer D, et al: Intermittent trimethoprim-sulfamethoxazole versus dapsone-pyrimethamine for the simultaneous primary prophylaxis of pneumocystis pneumonia and toxoplasmosis in HIV-infected patients. Ann Intern Med. 1995;122:755-761
162. Derouin F, et al: Synergistic activity of azithromycin and pyrimethamine or sulfadiazine in acute experimental toxoplasmosis. Antimicrob Agents Chemother. 1992;36:997-1001
163. Beaman MH, et al: Prophylaxis for toxoplasmosis in AIDS [Editorial]. Ann Intern Med. 1992;117:163-164
164. Havlir DV, et al: Prophylaxis against disseminated mycobacterium avium complex with weekly azithromycin, daily rifabutin, or both. N Engl J Med 1996;335:392-398
165. Pierce M, et al: A randomized trial of clarithromycin as prophylaxis against disseminated mycobacterium avium complex infection in patients with advanced acquired immunodeficiency syndrome. N Engl J Med 1996;335:384-391
166. Bartlett JA, et al: Lamivudine plus zidovudine compared with zalcitabine plus zidovudine in patients with HIV infection. Ann Intern Med. 1996;125:161-172
167. Collier AC, et al: Combination therapy with zidovudine and didanosine compared with zidovudine alone in HIV-1 infection. Ann Intern Med. 1993;119:786-793
168. Fishl MA, et al: Combination and monotherapy with zidovudine and zalcitabine in patients with advanced HIV disease. the NIAID AIDS Clinical Trials Group. Ann Intern Med. 1995;122:24-32
169. D'Aquila RT, et al: Zidovudine resistance and HIV-1 disease progression during antiretroviral therapy. Ann Intern Med.1995;122:401-408
170. D'Aquila RT, et al: Nevirapine, zidovudine, and didanosine compared with zidovudine and didanosine in patients with HIV-1 infection. Ann Intern Med. 1996;124:1019-1030
171. Neil MH, et al: Survival in HIV-infected patients who have received zidovudine: comparison of combination therapy with sequential monotherapy and continued zidovudine monotherapy. Ann Intern Med. 1996;124:1031-1038
172. Larder BA, et al: HIV with reduced sensitivity to zidovudine isolated during prolonged therapy. Science. 1989;243:1731-1734
173. Larder BA, et al: Potential mechanism for sustained antiretroviral efficacy of zidovudine-lamivudine combination therapy. Science. 1995;269:696-699

174. Mellors JW, et al: Prognosis in HIV-1 infection predicted by the quantity of virus in plasma. Science. 1996;272:1167-1170
175. Mellors JW, et al: Mutation in HIV-1 reverse transcriptase and protease associated with drug resistance. Int Antiviral News. 1995;3:8-15
176. Richman DD: HIV therapeutics. Science. 1996;272:1886-1888
177. Condra JH, et al: In vivo emergence of HIV-1 variants resistant to multiple protease inhibitors. Nature. 1995;374:569-571
178. Richman DD: Resistance, drug failure, and disease progression. AIDS Res Hum Retroviruses. 1994;10:901-905
179. Shirasaka T, et al: Emergence of HIV-1 variants with resistance to multiple dideoxynucleosides in patients receiving therapy with dideoxynucleosides. Proc Natl Acad Sci USA. 1995;92:2398-2402
180. D'Aquila RT: HIV-1 chemotherapy and drug resistance. Clinical and Diagnostic Virology. 1995;3:299-316

INDEX